Demons on the Couch

Demons on the Couch:

Spirit Possession, Exorcisms and the DSM-5

By

Michael J. Sersch

Cambridge Scholars Publishing

Demons on the Couch: Spirit Possession, Exorcisms and the DSM-5

By Michael J. Sersch

This book first published 2019. The present binding first published 2024.

Cambridge Scholars Publishing

Lady Stephenson Library, Newcastle upon Tyne, NE6 2PA, UK

British Library Cataloguing in Publication Data
A catalogue record for this book is available from the British Library

ISBN: 978-1-0364-3789-3
ISBN (Ebook): 978-1-5275-2415-6

"There are two equal and opposite errors we can fall into concerning demons. One is to disbelieve their existence. The other is to believe, and to feel an excessive and unhealthy interest in them." C.S. Lewis (1942, p. 9)

"A phenomenon cannot be observed unless the observer has a metaphor through which to see it."
(Schenk, 2001, p. 101)

"At its root, therapy derives from a word meaning 'to hold up, to support'. Therapy gives us the satisfaction of being useful... And often therapy does some good. Yet it can also feed our sense of self-importance, and inadvertently fuel our fear of futility. Therapy is not the same as healing."
(Norris, 2008, p. 141)

"Beware of stripping a patient who can't bear the chill of reality. And don't exhaust yourself by jousting with religious magic: you're no match for it. The thirst for religion is too strong, its roots too deep, its cultural reinforcement too powerful." (Yalom, 1989, p. 165)

CONTENTS

INTRODUCTION

Vomiting, profanity, levitation, blasphemy.

The images of demonic possession have infiltrated American culture, particularly in film. Much of this is due to the enduring popularity of the 1973 movie, *The Exorcist* (Blatty & Frieden, 1973) and the subsequent subgenre that the film helped create, although other scholars have addressed the cultural continuity of possession narratives going back to at least Biblical times (Levack, 2013).

I have begun to take my children on Fridays to a combined pizza parlor and video store, the only video store available in town. While browsing through their stacks of new releases, I am amazed at the number of films that involve a storyline of possession by demons or other spirits. A recent search of the website Internet Movie Database (IMDB, 2013) found over 200 titles when searching for the word "exorcism". I had recently written my thesis on this topic (Sersch, 2013) and had seen the phenomenon then, but it seems to have grown almost exponentially in the last several years. One aspect of this can be attributed to the conservative business approach within Hollywood; "if a project was successful, let us copy it until the theme no longer generates revenue". Using that model, the incredible success of *The Exorcist* (Blatty & Frieden, 1973) can help explain why, over 40 years later, the theme is still powerful. But that still leaves open the question as to why the theme of spirit/demonic possession is interesting to parts of the movie watching public, and has been so since the release of *The Exorcist*?

As Boggs has addressed (1996), themes from popular films tend to reproduce themselves, both among other films and also across society. Possession and subsequent exorcisms form one such theme in film. Rothman (1996) asked the rhetorical question, "Is God Really Dead in Beverly Hills?" when so much popular culture focuses upon the supernatural. Victoria Nelson argues in *Gothicka*: *Vampire Heroes, Human Gods and the New Supernatural* (2012) that with the steady disenchantment of the contemporary Western world, all that remains of the formerly sacred is the darkly supernatural. This includes possession stories, vampire romances and of course, zombies. This is often manifested in electronic media, of which people are consuming increasing amounts, not only of films but also television programs that include possession, such as *The Twilight Zone*, *The X-Files*, *Buffy the Vampire Slayer, and Supernatural,* as well as science fiction stories that include alien possession, such as the franchises of *Star Trek*, *Stargate* and *Dr. Who*, to name only a few (see Braak, 2015).

It is possible that what we are seeing is a form of post-modern spirituality. Hoyt (1978) quotes an unnamed film executive as claiming that themes like exorcisms in media satisfy an audience hungry for "mysticism, the supernatural, and the psychic. It's a kind of pop religion" (p. 4). Taylor (2007) notes that the desire to see the (pseudo) historic or supernatural creates a *frisson* within the individual; it is a nostalgic view of the past that is somehow more appealing and meaningful than modern life. Natoli (1994) has written rather poetically that, "We are haunted by what we cannot fully identify, by what we cannot make identical to what we already are, have, and know…Nothing is discovered; everything is rediscovered" (p. ix).

It has been reported that between 2000 and 2005, between 40% and almost 50% of the American public believed demonic possession was possible (www.whatstheharm.com), and Gallop (2015) has shown an increase in belief in the devil, from 55% of the American public in 1990 to 70% in 2007. This is interestingly around the same time that there is a noted steady decrease in a belief in God, from 96% in 1994 to 91% in 2011 and 86% in 2014 (Gallop, 2015). Geography affects these trends; Possamai (2015) notes that among Americans in the South, 59% report a belief in the possibility of possession, as compared with 48% of the general American population. Ruickbie (2012) cites 95% of respondents in the Ivory Coast who believe a person can be affected by witchcraft, whereas only 15% of those in Uganda responded similarly. There has even been a two-time Republican candidate for US presidential office in 2012 and 2016, governor of Louisiana Bobbi Jindhal, who has admitted to being involved in an exorcism while a college student, although that admission has also been politically costly (Dart, 2015).

Possession and exorcism are also an area that is easily mocked. The National Public Radio Show *Wait, Wait, Don't Tell Me* (2014) included a satirical story, as told by Roy Blount Jr., of an American southern pastor who had stated that "health food is satanic". In response, an area organic grocery store created "Healthy as Hell Week" and included an interview with a produce clerk dressed as a possessed beet (*Wait*…2014). It is worth noting that while the story is told humorously, there are plenty within the religious world that quickly attribute satanic influences to a wide variety of factors, as shall be shown in Chapter 3. The tendency to mock the phenomenon is also widespread: when I presented my initial findings in my graduate program, I was able to show a clip of a Saturday Night Live skit with Richard Pryor playing an exorcist trading "your mama" jokes with a young possessed girl. One of my heroes, the American Trappist monk

Thomas Merton (1915-1968), made light of area reports of possession immediately after his ordination to the priesthood (Mott, 1993). He later complained, "Certainly the complex business of being a 'personality' and exorcising the public demon it involves–all this is too much" (Mott, 1993, p. 524).

Jenny Lawson (2015) is a blogger who writes humorously of her struggles with mental health.

> Sometimes being crazy is a demon and sometimes the demon is me. . . I suppose we're all possessed in some way. Some of us with dependence on pills or wine. Others through sex or gambling. Some of us through self-destruction or anger or fear… My psychiatrist told me that when things get rough I should consider my battle with mental illness as if I were 'exorcising a demon" and I was like, 'Well, no wonder I'm failing so miserably. I'm shit at exercising.' Then she called me out for deflecting with humor, and explained: 'You are exorcising a demon. It's not something you can do alone. Some people do it with a priest and holy water. Some do it with faith. Some do it with chemicals and therapy. No matter what, it's hard.' 'And usually people end up with vomit on them,' I replied. (np)

Brave humor in the face of the challenges of personal transformation, in the battling of each individual demon, is the heart of what this text will attempt to provide.

Soon after *The Exorcist* book and film were released, a bestselling non-fiction book was written by a former Roman Catholic priest, Malachi Martin (1976), which told of six exorcisms in a graphic manner. Literature has addressed possession frequently; including such widely different authors as the Russian, Fyodor Dostoyevsky (1872, trans. 2009) and British authors such as William Shakespeare in the plays *Twelfth Night* (1623/2005), *A Comedy of Errors* (1623/2005), *Macbeth* (1623/2005), *Othello* (1622/2005), *King Lear* (1623/2005) and *King Henry V Part 1* (1623/2005). The latter play is now noted as having the possession scene, in which Joan of Arc beseeches demonic forces to come to her aid before her capture by the English, being penned by rival playwright Christopher Marlowe (Alberge, 2016). More recent English authors Aldous Huxley (1958, 1971) and William Golding (1971) also included possession narratives as a part of their writing. Further international authors with similar themes include Haruki Murakami (1994) from Japan, the Columbian Nobel Prize winner Gabriel Garcia Marquez (1995), the American authors Carole Muske-Dukes (2008) and Toni Morrison (1987) and the Italian author Umberto Eco (2011). Some use possession and exorcism as a powerful symbol in dealing with family dynamics and having multiple cultural identities, as does the Cuban American author Christina Garcia (1993). Furthermore, a subgenre of Japanese graphic novels known as "manga" frequently involves some form of demonic or other unwanted spiritual possession (Cuneo, 2001). For Kiev (1966), the experience of seeing a possession state is so moving for the audience, they collectively search for an explanation, using whatever categories are socially and culturally sanctioned. This may be one reason the trope is so often used in literature and in film.

Daniel Burke (2011) and Michael Cuneo (2001) have stated that the practice of exorcism has been steadily increasing in the last several decades. The Roman Catholic Church in the US has been making a concerted effort to increase the number of trained exorcists (Burke, 2011) although several years ago there were only 30 trained in the US (Koningisor, 2011). Protestant evangelicals, Pentecostals and fundamentalists have increased ministries involving exorcisms or deliverance prayers to drive away unwanted spiritual entities (Cuneo, 2001). Hoyt (1978) documents how the Anglican Church established guidelines for exorcisms in 1963 to respond to the increase in requests for the rite, and Levack (2013) notes that 1/3 of parishes in England had some form of deliverance ministry. Minority religious communities in the UK and the US, particularly immigrants and their children, have also brought exorcisms and spirit possession practices to further attention, as in the case of the young Hmong girl with epilepsy featured in *The Spirit Catches You and You Fall Down* (Fadiman, 1997). The situation of exorcism and child abuse among Nigerian immigrants to the UK was made into a novel by Christine Watson (2015b), due in part to her experience as a pediatric nurse seeing the increase in abuse among that population, which she attributes to the challenge of adaptation to a new culture (Watson, 2015a).

Cumo (2015) documents how there are at present three different organizations for those who are interested in the ministry of exorcism: the International Association of Exorcists or IAE (which is strictly for Roman Catholic priests, although it is not formally connected to the Vatican), the International Catholic Association of Exorcists or ICAE (which is open to Anglican, Gnostic, Orthodox and Catholic lay and priestly members), and the American Association of Exorcists (which was founded by a Baptist pastor and involves a level of licensing, see www.americanexorcist.com). Deslippe (2015) notes another school led by Pastor Bob Larson, the International School of Exorcism, although it appears that Pastor Larson, who is often wearing a Roman collar in spite of no listed denominational affiliation, may be more of a brand than an actual ministry. He appears to have an entire YouTube channel and each page of his website (www.boblarson.com) links to an opportunity to pay for the service.

The anthropologist Tanya Luhrmann (2005) has posited a theory labeled *absorption* as explaining the contemporary rise of possession, trance, and dissociative disorders. She argues that cultures always have some form of altered perception but the prevalence waxes and wanes over time. Contemporary culture needs, and is therefore allowing, a greater deal of both positive and negative dissociations within individual experiences as a way of coping with contemporary needs and stressors (see also Lewis, 2015b).

This text is not an attempt to prove or disprove controversial concepts like demonic possession; there are already books and articles that purport to either prove (Kiely & McKenna, 2007; Peck, 2005) or disprove (Cortes & Gatti, 1975; Shermer, 2003) the experience. Rather, I hope to build upon those who have already reported upon the phenomenon (Baglio, 2009; Cuneo, 2001; Goodman, 1988a, 1988b; Hoyt, 1978; Wilkinson, 2007) in order to better understand it. Furthermore, a number of mental health practitioners have directly addressed spirit possession among their clients (e.g. Bull, 2001; Bull, Ellason & Ross, 1998; Crabtree, 1997a; Isaacs, 2010; Kiev, 1966, 1973, 1979; Peck, 1995, 2005). In writing this book, I hope to answer why demonic possession has held a cultural fascination for over two millennia as well as how clinicians can successfully and ethically deal with patients who legitimately believe they are possessed by a spiritual force. There is also mounting evidence that integrating a patient/client's worldview into clinical practice, including their spirituality and faith practices, increases their likelihood of getting better (Lund, 2014), which is a position I am overtly advocating.

Understanding the Phenomenon

I must begin with the assumption that demonic possession is a phenomenon that some patients believe they experience. As stated in the most recent Diagnostic and Statistical Manual (DSM-5) of the American Psychiatric Association, under Dissociative Identity Disorder or DID (APA, 2013), possession is often a culturally sanctioned explanation for symptoms to which outside observers might ascribe different explanations. DID does not always translate well to other cultures, as Van Duijl, Cardeña and de Jong (2005) showed when comparing dissociative disorder understandings with traditional diagnoses in Uganda, particularly in regards to possession. We should not be limited solely to DID, however, as many other diagnoses can be understood by patients as due to spirit possession, including not only mental health concerns but also substance use and various physical ailments.

Because this text attempts to examine the phenomenological state of possession, it will use a variety of academic disciplines, including of course mental health fields like psychology and counseling theories, but also will include sociology, anthropology, literary and film theory, theology and the history of religions as well as the ever-evolving brain science. Such an approach has precedents, such as the historian Morris' (2011) examination of current Western hegemony. As he notes, while this approach allows for a breadth of vision, it is inherently limited, as no author can be expected to have a mastery of all the disciplines utilized. From a more subjective perspective, Quinones-Rosado (2010) has integrated mental health work among a diverse client population with an economic and political analysis of systems of oppression. His approach marries traditional therapy and social work with indigenous traditions native to the client, allowing the work of liberation to be unique and idiosyncratic. For an example of this integrative cross-disciplinary style within this subject, Khalifa and Hardie's (2005) research on Jinn possession among Islamic immigrants to the UK is an excellent example.

As a text that utilizes phenomenology, it is indebted to the original work of Hegel (1827/1968), who began the philosophical exploration of phenomenology, to be picked up by existential thinkers like Husserl (1900), Heidegger (1927/1968) and Frankl (1969, 1988). While Husserl (1900) helped to create the category of phenomenology, for him it was *a way of seeing* that led to transcendent truth about a *thing-in-itself* (Cairns, 1960). For existentialists, the phenomenon that is studied is wide-angled and tends to focus on a whole picture. For religious studies (James, 1995), phenomenology tends more toward examining specific rituals or beliefs, often from the perspective of those who are experiencing the particular phenomenon, a stance which has particular relevance for this study. And for others like Gabel (2013), phenomenology can be an act of not only academic importance but political and spiritual engagement, a way of looking at *The Other* that moves beyond metaphoric demonization toward an "I and Thou" relationship, in Martin Buber's terms (1970). Wolheim identifies that Buberian insight as a foundational insight in psychotherapy (2014).

All of this is a long way of stating that this is a book that looks at the phenomena of possession and exorcism as more than just pathology. The purpose of this text is to attempt an answer to the question, "*How can a culturally sensitive clinician treat a person who believes themselves to be possessed, in a manner that is both ethical and effective*?"

Layout of the Book

The book is laid out in such a manner that it can be read straight through or a reader may wish to skip to certain parts. The first section deals with a history of spirit possession in general and demonic possession in particular, from an ancient to a modern understanding. The second section is much more focused on issues of clinical concern; including the history of the diagnosis of Multiple Personality Disorder and the eventual change to Dissociative Identity Disorder (DID) in the DSM-5. It also looks at mental health approaches and religious understandings in the light of post-modernity. Finally, the third section is an exploration of how clinicians can appropriately and ethically handle clients who believe that they are possessed.

It will be noticed that while most of the book is written in the passive voice common with APA style, there will be moments of personal reflection. This break in the style is designed to highlight certain personal experiences. I apologize if it is distracting, but frankly I find the dry distance of APA to be a bit dull for a reader and as a writer. There is a question of the use of sources in such a text as this. Some existing literature is academic but may be rather old, such as Oesterreich's *Possession and Exorcism* (1930). Other writers on the subject tend toward the idiosyncratic, such as the colorful character Montague Summers (1926, 1958), a man who passed himself off as a Roman Catholic prelate and wrote in an antiquated manner about the subject, viewing himself as the last of the witch-hunters (Radl, 2012). As much as possible, this work will attempt to cast a wide net to include many writers in multiple fields in order to get a sense of perspective upon the subject.

SECTION 1

CHAPTER ONE

SPIRIT POSSESSION

Before looking at the phenomenon of demonic possession specifically, it is helpful to define spirit possession from a broad perspective. Possession is defined as a trance state that includes the loss of the individual's persona and social identity, which is replaced by an alien entity, usually spiritual or at least non-human (Bourguignon, 1976; Crapanzano & Garrison, 1977; Davies, 1995). Davies (1995), in quoting Oesterreich (1930), clarifies that the persona of the person possessed is not to be understood as a normally changing, dynamic part of the original person's self. Rather, this is a completely different persona, and is usually interacted with in the context as if they are another person (see also Lewis, 1986/2003). Persona, in this sense, should not be confused with other definitions, like those of C. G. Jung (1976) who views the persona as a "mask worn" allowing an individual the chance to function in the world.

Crabtree (1997a) identifies the pioneering American psychiatrist William James' (1842-1910) theory of personality as being "possessed by multiple selves" (p. 394), with various selves available depending upon the situation and the needs being addressed. Persona and personality are terms that carry multiple understandings, due in part to theoretical understanding; it is for this reason I will try and use the term *alters* or *multiples* to describe the personality as manifested in DID unless that alter is specifically understood to be a spirit.

Cohen (2008) makes a different distinction, between possession that is a replacement of the person (which she labels executive possession) and possession that leaves the personality alone but which brings illness or curses/bad luck (labeled as pathological possession). Crabtree (1997a) differentiates between *trance possessions*, which involve a separate entity being in control and often include amnesia for the person possessed and *lucid possession*, which occurs when the person is aware of and passively observes the possession. Mikles (2015) documents the universal frequency of spirit possession within storytelling traditions, including classical Greek epic poetry but continuing into contemporary Tibetan storytelling as well as West African *griot* traditions of bards.

Prothero (2010), in writing about the African diaspora religious traditions that stem from Yoruba practices, differentiates between those practices within this tradition and other possession narratives:

> Yoruba trance dancing is often referred to as spirit possession, but that is not quite right, since the *orisha* [possessing deity] possessed both the body and the spirit of the devotee. Every word, gesture, and movement of someone who had 'made the god' manifests the possessor rather than the possessed…The most common analogy, however, is to a rider 'mounting' a horse–an image that carries with it sexual connotations of a dominant male 'mounting' a submissive female. (p. 237)

Belief in possession extends to objects as well as persons, as the entire concept of hauntings and poltergeists shows. Numerous films have been made about items being possessed, such as dolls (Duppils, 2015c) or houses (Morehead, 2015d). There seems to be a special creative tension when safe possessions, such as a child's toy or the family home, are seen as somehow evil or dangerous, revealing a degree of personal and social anxiety.

Trance States

The ability to enter a trance state, however it is understood, is available to all societies, if not all people (Bourguignon, 1973; Crabtree, 1997b). It is seen by some as a key part of worship, including in the Christian traditions known as Pentecostal and Charismatic (Blumhofer, 2000; Cox, 1995; Cuneo, 2001; Goodman, 1988a; Quebedeaux, 1983), although there are others who argue that glossolalia, or speaking in tongues, should not be seen as a form of trance state (Werse, 2015b). Trance states are a common experience among African and Afro-Caribbean worshippers, both in traditional African practices (Goodman, 1988b; Stoller, 1989; Stoller & Olkes, 1987; Watters, 2011) and in overtly Christian Pentecostal forms in places like Brazil (Dawson, 2015). Numerous so called "primitive" societies engage in shamanistic trance states to deal with a variety of problems in the world, from illness to identifying animals for the hunt as well as other questions, such as divination (Kiev, 1966). In fact, Hale (2009) claims that there is not a time in the past or present when shamanistic practice has not been practiced. Luhrmann (2005) has argued that the process of trance is connected with the ability to vividly imagine what one wishes, and this skill can be heightened in certain people and in certain circumstances. Crabtree (1997a) and (2009) notes how in many alternative religious traditions in the West, such as neo-shamanism and Wicca, trance states are often a part of the religious practice (see for example Harner, 1980). Ezzy (2015) documents how in contemporary neo-pagan practice, especially among self-identified Heathens, ecstatic trance and possession by natural entities or spirits are common. While comparisons from ancient societies to modern practice can be tenuous, Hale (2009) has shown how cultural similarities are often looked at in anthropology and archeology as a way to give a sense of how pre-historic practices were performed and understood.

Kiev (1973) describes the techniques of the introduction of the trance state by "repetitive bodily movements, reduced sensory stimulation, exhaustion, hypoglycemia, and physical stress" (p. 29). Hale (2009) notes that the use of music is common in bringing about a trance state. A person achieving this trance state may do so via the use of intoxicating hallucinogenic substances such as the ayahuasca plant in the Brazilian rainforest (Dawson, 2015). The trance itself carries with it a degree of risk, as Balikci (1967) documents an indigenous Netsilik shaman named Anaidjuq whose possessing spirit would reportedly pull on his genitals.

It is worth noting that not all trance states result in spirit possession. In writing about a Hindu healer who worked in the States, Woodward (2016) writes, "When she turned her head I noticed that her eyes were turned upward, much like the eyes of exorcists I'd seen in Africa during a trance" (p. 268). The famous scholar of religion Mercia Eliade (1907-1986) as cited by Harvey (2015), in fact separates shaman trance states from possession. As Crabtree (1997b) has noted, trance states occur with frequency in daily life (such as the mild hypnotic effects of windshield wipers on the driver of a car). They can also be understood as an aspect to all understanding: there is a relationship trance where one sees the beloved in a way that others do not, a family trance, and a social trance. Satoh, et al. (1996) even document how a trance state can develop with both a customer and a salesperson in the midst of door-to-door sales. Crabtree (1997b) recognizes the necessity of many of those "trances" but also encourages clinical work to "break the spell" of a variety of trances in order to live more authentically. This approach seems very similar to Transaction Analysis (Berne, 1964) in the examination of the "games" that people use. Kirby (2006) argues that the media, especially electronic media, help to create a "pseudo-modern" trance that robs people of intellectual originality. I can attest to seeing such a trance when my young children become engrossed in the consumption of electronic media.

However, the effects of acute religious trance states can include incredible creativity among those who are engaged in the trance. As Goodman (1988b) states:

> I have heard hardworking, taciturn Mayan peasants, who in ordinary life had a difficulty uttering two coherent sentences in public, bringing forth

> poetry of surpassing beauty in ecstasy. Japanese religious leaders write truly enormous volumes of religious thought, again in poetic form, while possessed by their deity. . . And the pronouncements of demons, thought to speak from the mouths of the possessed, have been quoted by emperors and popes. (p. 9)

The trance state associated with spirit possession can also be associated with demonic or unclean spirits, which does not eliminate the chance for creative output (Spiegel, et al., 2011).

Certain cultures place a strong emphasis upon trance states. Uganda, for example, has experienced years of conflict that included forces initially led by Alice Auma (1956-2007), an illiterate woman from the Acholi people who are predominate in Northern Uganda (Sagert, 2015). In 1986 she began to channel "Lakwenda", a spirit she identified as belonging to a deceased Italian army officer after one of her tribespeople was overthrown from governmental leadership. She led the Holy Spirit Movement which militarily fought the government until its defeat one year later. Her troops were said to be in a trance when fighting, as well as being ceremonially covered in oil before battle to protect them from bullets and they carried stones believed to turn into grenades. These ritual magical ideas seem similar to the Native American Ghost Dance of the late 19th century, when fighters would wear tunics to protect themselves from bullets and it was believed that the White settlements would be somehow removed from the Earth (Brown, 2001), and the Boxer Rebellion in China (Thompson, 2001) at the turn of the 20th century, when forces that engaged in spirit possession by Taoist and Buddhist Deities fought against the 8 nations attempting the colonial takeover of the mainland.

A relative of Auma, Joseph Kony, reorganized the remaining forces into the Lord's Resistance Army. He identified a number of possessing entities, including "Major Bianca", "King Bruce" and "Silver". The Lord's Resistance Army has displaced over one million people and forced thousands of youths into their services, either militarily or as sex slaves. Ugandan possession states have been studied in a variety of papers, including interviews with those who were fighters in the uprisings as well as those who were displaced by the fighting (e.g. Neuner, et al.; Reis, 2013; Van Duijl, Cardeña, & de Jong, 2005; Van Duijl, Kleij, & de Jong, 2013; Van Duijl, Kleijn, de Jong, 2014; van Duijl, et al., 2013). It is interesting that possession is reported among both the fighters and those who were forced to flee from the conflicts.

Shamanic Practices

Morris (2011) has theorized, based upon studies of the early cave paintings in France and other places, that shamanism may have been the earliest expression of religion. Weiner (2011) points to the overlap between the roles the shaman helps to play within tribal societies and contemporary mental health care, including diagnoses, medication interventions, behavioral modifications, and supportive listening. Young (2018) claims that the role of shaman is often held by women, at least earlier in the historic record, although the literature includes significant male and female shamans as well as shamans who cross clear gender boundaries. Hale (2009) points to the fact that in tribal society the shaman is the only role that is exclusive, all other behaviors may be gender-based but could be performed by anyone within the tribe (such as hunting, building structures, cooking, etc.). This stands in direct contrast to the specialization that characterizes contemporary societies. While Levi-Strauss documents a shaman who in all other ways is like other tribal members (1967), it is clear that shamans often stand somewhat apart from the rest of the tribe in some way. Ambrose (1996) cites Crazy Horse's friend in the Oglala tribe Pretty One aka Woman Dress (birth and death dates unknown), who worked as a shaman as well as being a *winkte*, a person born a man but who dressed as a woman and had sexual relationships with both men and women. On the other hand, Kehoe (2000) cautions against generalized approaches across cultures when looking at shamanistic practice, viewing this tendency among scholars as a racist use of the Noble Savage myth. While shamans appear to have an important role in many societies, the role does carry some risk. In looking at pottery from the pre-Incan societies in Peru, one artifact shows shamanic characters being devoured by vultures. This has led to the theory that these were unsuccessful in their healing rites as the shaman appears to be alive while being consumed (Hale, 2009).

Levi-Strauss (1967) discusses previous research done by Boas (1930) in explaining the autobiographic writings of Quesalid (birth and death dates unknown), a Kwakwaka'wahk First Nation shaman from the Vancouver area. Quesalid began to be initiated into shamanic practices both within his tribe and a neighboring tribe. He was disturbed at the use of sleight-of-hand tricks, such as hiding a bloody piece of down inside the mouth, a form of psychic surgery (removing the sickness from the ill person), or driving hidden nails within the shaman's dwelling which appeared to cause a sacred rattle to levitate in the air. He soon challenged another shaman to a "healing duel" as a way of discovering some more illusions, and was more successful in convincing the suffering person of his power. This reportedly led the other shaman to go mad and leave the village. However, as he continued to practice, he began to move toward a position of recognizing the healing power of rituals while affirming the inherent trickery in the practice.

Prevalence of Possession

We know that possession belief was widespread in the ancient world. The skeptical philosopher Larry Shapiro refers to possession throughout history as an example of "negative miracles" in the sense that they appear to be supernatural in a generally non-helpful manner (2016). Exorcisms by Jesus are detailed in the Gospel accounts (Davies, 1995). A long catalogue of illnesses and their demonic origins (as well as identifying angels who can counteract their effects) is used in the Gnostic text *The Apocryphon of John,* dating to before 185 CE (Wisse, 1988).

Bourguignon (1976) surveyed the work of anthropologists who examined 488 cultures, and discovered that 437 had beliefs in altered states of consciousness (ASC) including trance, possession or both, which is 90 per cent of the surveyed cultures. This left 51 (or 10%) of the surveyed cultures without a belief in an ASC like spirit possession. Ellenberger (1970) noted no belief in possession among certain tribes in the Philippines, the Malay Peninsula or among the Aboriginal people of Australia. In commenting on these findings of Bourguignon (1976), Davies (1995) points out that it is possible that the people in those cultures may have not shared their belief in ASC with the anthropologists studying them, so the actual figures of belief in ASC may be higher. He writes:

> Possession is not a fiction, not a pretense, not a kind of folk belief. Possession is a powerful psychophysiological experience that is so widespread in human cultures that the potential for the possession experience is part of the genetic inheritance of all people. To put it bluntly, if you do not occasionally become possessed it is because you have not placed yourself in circumstances where the achievement of the possession state is possible. (Davies, 1995, p. 25)

Goodman (1988b), when writing about Bourguignon's findings (1976), notes that spirit possession is culture-specific. Cultural beliefs are not static and do change, as documented by Dien, Alexander and Napier (2008) when looking at the length of time and education attained among immigrant communities in the UK. In a study in the US among inpatient residents in a psychiatric hospital, a high number reported a belief in possession and some had engaged in exorcisms to help with their symptoms (Ross, Schroeder & Ness, 2013).

Goodman (1988b) further notes that belief in something like spirit possession necessitates a belief in individuals having a spirit that can be possessed by an alien force, which she calls "soul theory". However, this does not include experiences of delusions, which may occur among people who ordinarily do not focus upon supernatural forces. Crabtree (1997b) has argued that possession states, like other "inner mind experiences" (p. 104) such as paranormal phenomena, are particularly difficult for Western people due to the widespread dismissal of the soul theory. Crabtree (1997a; 1997b) further advances that it is not necessary for the practitioner to have any belief in the objective reality of the patient's experiences or even subscribe to the "soul theory" themselves, only to understand that it is meaningful for the patient.

Common Possession Understanding in Africa

Goodman (1988b) separates spirit possession from demonic possession by stating that while spirit possession is intended (as in the acts of a shaman), demonic possession is unintended and unwanted, a distinction that is helpful but not used in much of the literature and as such, will not be followed in this text. Goodman (1988b) further separates the African understanding of possession and exorcism from the Eurasian ones, which are found in the Indian subcontinent, Asia, Europe and large parts of the Americas, although it is seen among the African diaspora due to the history of the slave trade. Within the African concept, possession may be by a positive or negative deity. Negative possession is sometimes by a ghost of the departed or a spirit and is treated with an exorcism that mimics a burial and subsequent rebirth. This is the style used in Haiti, Brazil and other areas with a strong African connection (Brown, 1991; Harrison, 2000).

Zora Neal Hurston (1891-1960), a novelist and anthropologist who was active in the Harlem Renaissance of African American culture in the 1920s (Varlack, 2015), traveled to Haiti and described the rites involved in zombification as well as spirit possession in her book *Tell My Horse* (1938). Contemporary Ethiopia has had a reported 66 per cent of the population witness a form of exorcism (Lloyd, 2015a). This breaks down to 74 per cent of the Christian community (which includes the ancient Ethiopian Orthodox Church as well as contemporary Protestants), 44 per cent of the Egyptian Muslim community, and many who identify with one of the dominant traditions while also being involved in the Zar practices that are described later in this text (Lloyd, 2015a). In post-war Mozambique, the percentage of surveyed participants who reported being possessed was 18.6%, with 5.6% reporting more than one spirit as the possessor (Igreja, et al., 2010). Schmidt

(2015a) documents how throughout areas bordering the Atlantic Ocean, communities of the African diaspora practice variations of these sacred spirit possessions with regional differences. Leo Africanus (1494-1544?), whose family fled Islamic Spain due to the *Reconquista* and subsequently traveled widely in northern Africa, reported on Muslim exorcists who would call upon the name of the spirit and ask how it entered the possessed person. When unsuccessful in the exorcism, they would then attribute the possession to the will of Allah (Hoyt, 1978).

Lloyd (2015) states that a belief in possession by ancestors is often the explanation offered for sickness throughout much of the world. This is reported to be common among the Zulu, Xhosa, and Swazi people of southern Africa, but it has expanded to other tribes and the white community as well. The role of a diviner, who is possessed by an ancestral spirit and reveals the cause of the illness, is often reserved for women or gay men. Newell (2015), in examining the phenomena of trepanning, or creating a whole in the skull, does address the common belief that this ancient practice was often to address illnesses, although in truly ancient remains we can often only speculate as to why the procedure was performed given there is no written record. This practice is satirized in the trilogy *His Dark Materials* by Philip Pullman (1995, 1997, 2000), where one of the parallel universes includes frequent trepanation.

Eurasian Possession Understandings

Within the Eurasian model, possession can be by many entities, including ghosts (Kiely & McKenna, 2007) and in Islamic cultures, Jinns or what used to be called in the West "genies", such as in Aladdin (see Khalifa & Hardie, 2005). Within Pentecostal communities, a wide variety of ailments like lust or addiction (Cuneo, 2000; Kraft, 2010) can be seen as a form of possession. Eurasian possession is often seen as negative and almost always unwanted, except in a few cases reported of those associated with occult practices (see, for example, Martin, 1976). A specific example is cited by Hanley & Brown (2014), who examined postnatal Arabic women who described possession by Jinns; their descriptions of sadness, anxiety, and physical malaise match a Western medical understanding of post-partum depression. Hinduism includes positive possessions by deities and negative possession leading to a variety of illnesses (Fibiger, 2015). In a recent study in Turkey of 618 women, over 2% reported a personal belief that they had been possessed in their life (Sar, Alioğlu & Akyüz, 2014).

A personal situation may help to explain Eurasian possession, as I understand it. My neighbor is a Hmong shaman, as was her husband. The

Hmong are a people who had lived primarily in Laos as subsistence hunters and farmers, practicing a spirituality focused on animistic and shamanistic practices. They joined US forces fighting against the Laotian government in the Vietnam War, an expansion of the war which was not well known in the US (Donnelly, 1994). After the fall of Saigon, many left for Thailand where they lived in refugee camps until some were able to immigrate to the US, a difficult process as subsequent generations attempt to hold onto important cultural beliefs while also adjusting to post-modern American life (Fadiman, 1997). After my neighbor's husband had passed away she found herself in a period of prolonged grief and bereavement. Unable to get out of her dark space, the family invited another shaman to the home as well as her clan and neighbors. This fits with a solid rule within shamanistic practice, as noted by Hale (2009), that the healing can only be done by a shaman to others, a shaman cannot bring healing upon him/herself. An exorcism was performed so that the ghost of her deceased husband would leave her. She was then expected to do the cleanup from the gathering, which was substantial as both a hog and a cow were butchered in the backyard. (Blood was literally flowing down our shared alley, but as I got to enjoy some of the feasting, I was not too upset.) The expectation of the (formerly) possessed person to do the work after the Hmong healing ceremony has also been cited in DuBois (2009), and at the gathering it was explained to me that this helps her to re-enter the community.

Signs of Possession

What does possession look like? The classic Roman Catholic definition holds that the possessed can speak other languages not otherwise known, possess superhuman strength, and have knowledge beyond the person (Midelfort, 2005). Burke (2011) notes that using the formal Catholic definition results in very few instances of demonic possession being found, in spite of the fact that Catholic exorcisms are steadily increasing. In almost none of the contemporary texts reviewed in this study can these symptoms be observed or verified, they are often not even reported (e.g. Baglio, 2009; Cuneo, 2001; Peck, 2005; Wilkinson, 2007). What is reported in contemporary reports includes some banal experiences, an unnamed exorcist is quoted as saying that one possessed person repeated "Hickory Dickory Dock" (Koningisor, 2011) while another included coughing fits (Baglio, 2007).

Some traditions within Islam have included physical illness and mental illness (including the hearing of voices) as symptoms of possession (Eneborg, 2015). Levack (2013) has shown that the classical definition within Catholicism was not always strictly observed and differed from many Protestant traditions which, at least among Calvinists, tended to emphasize personal sinfulness. American Puritans observed a number of possessions associated with witchcraft that included fits, seizures, and hallucinations (Demos, 2008). Cited texts by Levack (2013) include commonly observed phenomena such as muscle rigidity and/or flexibility, pain, convulsions, levitation, swelling, vomiting, catatonia, and immoral gestures and actions including revulsion at sacred items and blasphemy. The tendency to vomit foreign objects is often associated with extreme self-harming behaviors and, according to Walsh (2014), usually is seen among the very psychologically ill as a coping strategy, such as prisoners who then are sent to the infirmary. While parallels in this category over vast time-frames and among culturally different people might be hard to draw, it is reasonable to assert that the consumption of foreign objects has historically been a sign of extreme distress.

In an interview with Malcom Poussaint, a Benin emigrant who works as a traditional exorcist among the African Diaspora in London, Tahir (2005) documents behavior among children which might trigger parents to seek out Poussaint's rituals: "running around, screaming, making noise, acting abnormally, hitting things, hitting people, jumping on the sofa" (n.p.). (As a parent of two small children, it is hard to imagine that my own children do not meet these criteria at some times on most days.) The ritual that Poussaint uses includes having the parents hold the child while he and they recite prayers, often after the child is bathed. The child is also anointed with oil and often all those who are gathered enter into a trance state, aided by Poussaint's drumming.

Possession and the Body

Bourguignon (1976) differentiated between spirit possession (the replacement of the self with another) and possession belief (which attributes an illness or other physical symptom to the influence of the spirit). Possession has long been connected with physical as well as psychological disease. The figure of Zoroaster (also known as Zarathustra, circa 1500? BCE) is widely considered a shaman and exorcist and his influence included significant use of these rituals in Persia (Hoyt, 1978). Hoyt (1978) documents how all illness for ancient Egypt was tied to possession by evil spirits or Gods, and the role of exorcist was often combined with doctoring. A frequent type of ritual would include bread, beer, incense, and a statue of the god invoked. A stela (a stone inscribed by hieroglyphs) was discovered in a temple of the god Khonsu. It claims to date from the famous Pharaoh

Ramses II (circa 1303-1213 BCE) but was more likely created around 500 BCE. The stela tells of the possession of a foreign princess by a demon and her eventual healing when the statue of the god was transported, a story that seems to convey a sense of the power of the Egyptian Empire and Gods (Mansen, 2015). Duppils (2015b) notes how cultures as different as the Navajo (2015a) in the American Southwest and Sweden through history identify illnesses as caused by contact with spiritual forces.

A frequent example of possession stated in the literature is the confusion of epilepsy and possession. One of the miraculous exorcisms documented in the Gospel of Luke (9:39) is of an epileptic man. In a current study of school teachers and university students in Saudi Arabia, 40% and 50% respectively reported that epilepsy (in Arabic, *saraa*) is due to possession by "jinn" (Obeid, et al., 2012). As shown by Islam and Campbell (2014), this is not inherent in Muslim thought nor is it endorsed in the Quran, and thus it is more likely a symptom of a cultural belief. This association does not only occur in the Kingdom of Saudi Arabia, Baxendale (2003) documents how it is also common in Western film. This combination of epilepsy and possession is ancient, going back to the Greeks and it continued even after the widespread adoption of the bodily humor theory of Hippocratic physicians (Scull, 2015).

Nakken and Brodtkorb (2011) hypothesize that epilepsy accounts for a larger amount of religious experience and writing than has previously been thought. Examples abound, including Salzman's (2001) novel *Lying Awake*, about a contemporary nun who is emotionally shattered to discover her visions of the divine were related to a temporal lobe tumor which is causing seizures. Kugel (2011) speculates that the theory that religious states (either of the divine or demonic) as stemming from temporal lobe seizures, such as those that occur in epilepsy, may have the relationship inverted; what the person with epilepsy is experiencing is a window into the spiritual world, or at least another experience of reality.

Hoyt (1978), who appears to believe in possession states in general, points to the exorcism of two boys, Theobald and Joseph Burner. The boys lived in the Alsace region between France and Germany and in 1869 underwent an exorcism, although the writer clearly felt their symptoms were likely undiagnosed epilepsy. It is interesting that a stone column was reportedly erected to remember their "liberation from possession" (p. 59) in a region that has historically been such a sight of territorial conflict. I could not find any evidence of the column still standing.

Worldviews

The mid-century theologian R. Richard Niebuhr (1962, 1999) theorized that there are four main worldviews: mechanical, magical, malevolent, and malleable. Of the four, the mechanical is the only one that categorically eliminates the "soul theory". It is also the approach most closely associated with modernity and the scientific worldview (Greenblatt, 2011; Morris, 2011). Greenblatt (2011) associates the success of the Western world with the scientific worldview, the mechanical approach that dismisses the "soul theory" and consequently, the possibility of an outside force possessing that soul. Given this mechanical presumption, any person who reports being possessed by an outside spirit becomes labeled as mentally ill (Spiegel, et al., 2011). However, this is but one of the existing worldviews.

It ought not to be presumed that Western psychological insights are exclusive, or even superior. It has long been noted that schizophrenia and other forms of psychosis appear to have much in common with religious experiences; including visions/hallucinations, a focus on the divine and demonic, and a sense of time and perception that differs from the norm. Burton (2015) states that both religious experiences and psychosis include activity in the right hemisphere of the brain. As Watters (2011) has argued, when looking at the results of the World Health Organization's study of recovery rates of schizophrenia (Hopper & Wanderling, 2000), societies that have a strong belief in spiritual forces affecting a person's mental health are more effective than Western medical approaches in dealing with persistent mental illnesses. Some anthropologists, such as Michael Taussig, have suggested that Western approaches toward possession act as a form of colonization (Cumo, 2015b). Every other culture has an understanding of the human condition, often using different worldviews (Ivey, D'Andrea, & Ivey, 2012). Carroll (2014) states:

> Yet moderns make a mistake by dismissing the long-ago-conjured images of space, time, origins, personified forces, and fate as mere naiveté. An assumption of the superiority of our more critically considered worldview may lead us to miss the ingenious character of the old imaginings as sensitive penetrations to an impressive depth of the perennial mysteries of existence. (p 86)

Western approaches to mental health and illness may be dominant due to Western cultural hegemony. However, current cultural and economic superiority from Western societies should not be presumed to be preordained, everlasting, or a given (Morris, 2011). For example, China's economic growth is neither based upon Western values nor presumptions, but it is quickly becoming the world's largest economic force (*Economist*, 2012a). Brain scans have shown that people from China and other Asian cultures have different ways of seeing the world, their brains light up in other patterns that are different from the tendency of Western brains (Ivey, D'Andrea, & Ivey, 2012; Morris, 2011). Fox writes, "One becomes 'sick' or 'crazy' in a well-defined, cultural way…Primitive societies and religious healing groups often have the edge on hospitals in that they more often incorporate the sick person into the society and indeed often utilize the sickness in some cultural sphere" (1967, pp. 255-256). This does not prove the "soul theory", the possibility of spirit or demonic possession, or any sense of cultural superiority; it does however point to the fact that the world is experienced by each person mediated through both numerous idiosyncratic and socially ordained ways.

Anthropologists like Elms (1970) have pointed out that societies (including distinct counter-cultures) can collectively believe items that otherwise sane persons would reject. White (2006) rather helpfully clearly indicates that while contemporary society tends toward a post-modern understanding, persons may either be operating from a pre-modern, modern, or post-modern worldview. When approaching a client, from whatever culture or counter-culture they are from, it is important to remember their unique and personal experiences of the world. As Spiegel, et al. (2011) have noted, a patient's belief in spirit or demonic possession does not necessitate that the therapist holds the same belief, only that the practitioner respects such a belief as valid from the worldview of the patient.

CHAPTER TWO

HISTORY OF SPIRIT POSSESSION AND EXORCISM

Possession

The term possession carries within it a sense of metaphor, as the spirit *possesses* a person in the same way that an army *possesses* territory. Gray (1959), in writing about men on the battlefield, described their behavior as being like they were possessed by a demon. Spirit possession appears very early in the written record, and as Verter (2000) noted, spirit is an inclusive term, implying no inherent value. Early Greek texts like Homer's *Iliad* (trans. 1999) and *Odyssey* (trans. 1999) have numerous characters being possessed by one of the Olympian Gods (Porter, 2002). Kiev (1972) claimed that in the Classical Greek world, an oracle that was in a trance state due to possession by a God was held in the highest regard, although there were some forms of possession that were viewed ambiguously. These would include sexual infatuation (possession by Eros) or drunkenness (possession by Dionysus). There were also some forms of possession which were negative, which increasingly became associated with demons or other evil spirits (see Meggitt, 2015). Hale (2009) has shown how Greek religious practice often included visits to oracle sites, which were usually located over volcanic regions whose waters had mild hallucinogenic effects, allowing a prophet to speak in the voice of Apollo while in a trance. It should be noted that the oracles tended to be vague, allowing for various interpretations (Jacob, 2015a). Within the Greek world, a person may be harassed by evil spirits, such as the Furies, who often required a sacrifice such as when Orestes had to chop off a finger to have them abandon him (Kugel, 2011).

Exorcism

The term exorcism comes from *exorkizein*, the Greek for oath (Kiely & McKenna, 2007). The term was often used in a simple way with prayers for a meal, which in Christian rites came to be used over communion vessels

(Brock & Parker, 2008) as well as integrated into the blessing of water and of salt (Kustron, 2015). The first known written exorcism is the Hindu text *AtharvaVeda,* which was written between 1500 BCE (as claimed by Laycock, 2015a) and 2000 BCE, although the oral source is probably much older (Kiely & McKenna, 2007). Early Hindu texts often have demonic characters, such as the antagonist Ravana in the *Ramayana* (dated anywhere from 500 BCE to 200 BCE). In the text, Ravana must be defeated by a human, necessitating the deity Vishnu to become incarnated as Rama in order to establish a Utopian state and thereby legitimizing the existing power structure, or so argues Malik (2014). Hinduism has long allowed for a variety of possession states and various forms of exorcisms depending upon the caste of the person possessed. This is a practice that continues to the present day (Fibiger, 2015). It has been said that the very act of worship within a Hindu temple includes a sense of the temple and the statue of the God inside as being positively possessed. The statue of the deity is woken, bathed, fed, and then bedded as a part of the daily activities (Freeman, 2003).

Dein and Samad Illaiee (2009) document how many ailments in the ancient Sumerian Empire were attributed to the forces of evil spirits. Hoyt (1978) cites how Babylonian rituals included nearly constant exorcisms in the cultic center of Eridu. These rituals included calling upon the demon by a long recitation of known names, then placing the possessed upon a bed and sprinkling them with water. Notice how similar this ritual is to the filmed version of *The Exorcist* (Blatty & Friedken, 1973), which was made several millennia later. Occasionally animals were brought into the ritual so the departing spirits could possess another life. (This is also found in one of the synoptic Gospel stories, the *Gerasene demoniac*, see Matt. 12:45, Mark 5:11, Luke 8:2.) The theme of fear of the demonic and the power of folk practice in the Mesopotamian world can be seen in the prevalence of magic bowls found with Jewish, Christian, Manichean, and Mandean prayers inscribed in order to capture spirits, dating from the fifth to the eight century CE (Barnes, 2015).

Morris (2011) points to early Chinese examples in writing, including a nobleman who had an exorcism as part of dealing with a broken leg. Morris (2011) further argues that one of the reforms brought about by Confucius (see Analects 6:20, trans. 1995) was the limiting of exorcisms when ritual emphasis was instead placed on the veneration of ancestors (for a similar reading without a reference to exorcisms, see Eliade, trans. 1982). Hardy (2014) documents the common use of exorcisms in early Doaist practice. During the Han dynasty in China (206 BCE-220 CE), exorcisms by a shaman or a Confucian or Doaist priest would have been common, and often included animal sacrifice (Scull, 2015). Exorcism was incorporated into Tibetan Buddhism with the symbols of the cleaver and the cutting board being common, signifying both battling demons and cutting through ignorance (Kiely & McKenna, 2007). There are stories that the mother of Siddhartha, the historic Buddha, was herself an exorcism (Hoyt, 1978). There are some traditions within Islam, such as Zar, that include asking another spiritual being to displace a negative possession by a demon or jinn (Eneborg, 2015), as well as the Gnawa in Morocco, who believe Jinn possession can lead to the power to heal others (Jacob, 2015b). Pye (2014) notes that exorcism of water continued into the early medieval period as a preparation for trial by ordeal.

Frank and Frank (1991) note the similarities in healing rituals from exorcisms to modern-day psychotherapy in that, 1) the healer is socially santioned, 2) the person who is suffering has a belief in the power of the process, and 3) the contacts between the healer and the sufferer are structured with a goal of changing the lived experience of the sufferer. Gettis (1976) builds upon an earlier version of Frank's work to directly make the metaphoric connection of psychotherapy as exorcism, a theme which is also found in Thomason (2008).

Demon

Biblical uses of the term "demon" (in Latin, *daemon*) are somewhat difficult to establish as the word is a Greek term, so it would not have appeared in the original Hebrew writings. However, the influence of demons was a significant aspect of Zoroastrian belief, and it is believed to have been a major influence of Israel's religious community through the influence of the Babylonian captivity, which was ended by the conquest of Babylon by Persian forces who followed Zoroastrian practices in the 6th century BCE (Guiley, 2009). Hebrew thus does not have a specific word for demons but uses a variety of terms. Murphy (2015b) cites, for example, how in Leviticus Chapter 16 there is the famous ritual of the "scapegoat". On the Day of Atonement (Yom Kippur), two goats are identified in the Israelite encampment, one for "The Lord" (YHWH), which will be sacrificed, and another for "Azazel", which will be driven into the desert. There is significant scholarly debate about the root of the word "Azazel", as it could be a combination of the word "goat" (*ez*) and the word "to go away" (*azal*). However, the term quickly became associated with a specific demonic entity that makes later appearances in non-Canonical apocalyptic literature.

Kaplan (2012) notes that the origin of the Greek word "demon" comes from *daiein*, meaning "to distribute", as in spiritual entities that followed the wishes of the Gods on people's destinies. The term demon (Greek *daimon* or *daimonion*) was used by Socrates (Plato, trans. 1997) when crediting his ideas to his personal *daimon* (Baglio, 2009). This concept seems to be similar to a guardian angel, the soul, or even an inner voice. It should be noted that Aristotle (trans. 1984) denied the existence of demons. According to Cardin (2015a), Plato's student Xenocrates (395-314 BCE) differentiated between good daimons (*eudaimones*) and bad ones (*kakodaimones*). The older understanding of an inner voice began to be encouraged in the writings of Carl Jung (Cardin, 2015a). The concept of *daimon* has continued to influence several contemporary mental health theorists, including the existential humanist Rollo May (1970) and the Jungian James Hillman (1991), who advocate clients to re-engage with their personal *daimons* in order to integrate their whole self.

It does not appear that the word demon itself entered into English usage until the Benedictine Revival of the 11th century CE, when more Latin and Greek words entered the language (Lerer, 2008). The term demon evolved in Christian thought to become an exclusively evil spirit, a fallen angel (Russell, 1972, 1977). However, most religious traditions, including Hindu, Buddhist, Muslim and various Native American tribes, have morally ambiguous spirit forces (Verter, 2000). In the memoir by the Dakota (Sioux) Indian writer Zitkala-Sa (1921/1985), the author documents how belief in the devil was brought through the missionary efforts, including Native American boarding schools. Islam views demons, jinn (or djinn) and even Satan as ambiguous or incompetent, certainly evil but ineffective, or at least not as strong as viewed in Christianity (Armstrong, 2002). Russell (1972) claims the term *devil* comes from the Latin for *diablus*, originally the Greek *diaballein*, which meant to slander.

Dissociation

Dissociation, a psychiatric symptom for handling psychological trauma characterized by a continuum of behaviors all characterized by a detachment from the present, can be found across cultures and eras. However, there is evidence that it is especially common among some populations, such as Latinos (Lewis-Fernandez, et al., 2010), and in areas with a high incidence of conflicts, for example Uganda (Neuner, et al., 2012). In both of these examples, cultural schemas as well as the prevalence of trauma (both personal and at the social level) contribute to the manifestation of individuals with dissociation. In the newest edition of the DSM (APA, 2013), clinicians are encouraged to differentiate between "possessed state" and "non-possessed state" experiences of dissociation when looking at DID, although there is no differential diagnosis or differing clinical criteria (i.e. number) for the two. It is also stated as important that the experience of possession (or other disassociation) is impairing a person's normal activities and is not a normal part of a cultural or clinical practice. I take this to mean that while my Hmong neighbor's experience of bereavement is placed within her cultural schema of possession necessitating an exorcism, she could still have had a dissociation diagnosis. This diagnosis may not have meant much to her, but she was experiencing distress over her grieving. However, when she works as a shaman herself and goes into an ASC to do her work, that does not warrant a DID diagnosis.

Dollar (2015) has written about JZ Knight, a woman who had reached a degree of fame after being mentioned by the actor Shirley MacLaine in her book *Dancing in the Light* (1985) and in an appearance in the film *What The [bleeb] Do We Know?* (Arntz, Chasse & Vicente, 2004). Knight enters into dissociative trances and speaks with the voice of a spirit named Ramtha, who is claimed to have conquered Atlantis. Dollar (2015) notes how independent medical studies of Knight show a distinct difference in heart rate and other body functions when she has dissociation versus when she is Knight, a phenomenon that is common among people with DID, although in this case Knight has made millions from her trance state as opposed to experiencing impairment in daily functioning.

Possession in the Hebrew and Christian Scriptures

While visions and dreams are common in the Bible (Kiev, 1973), there is very little in the Hebrew Scriptures about spirit possession and only one example of an exorcism, and that is in a text which is not considered canonical by many branches of Christianity. However, Borg (2001) has stated that the books of the Prophets are written as if the authors are possessed by the spirit of God, a mystical tradition that appears in a modified form throughout mystical Judaism in the concept of the *ibbur*, where a holy man is "impregnated" with the spirit of a deceased teacher (Lior, 2015b).

Negative effects are sometimes, especially in the earlier writings, attributed to the power of negative spirits, often at the behest of God. This would include Judges Chapter 9 when YWHW sends an evil spirit (in Hebrew, a *ruah ra'ah*) to the judge Abimelech (maybe more accurately labeled a warlord, see Murphy, 2015a). When the possessed Abimelech flees from the city of Shechem, a revolt ensues, which is ended only through the execution of the judge/warlord by a large stone falling on his head.

Further negative effects plague King Saul, whose depression and violent moods are attributed to an evil spirit in I Samuel, Chapter 16.

The Book of Tobit is considered Deuterocanonical (literally second canon, or not containing the same degree of authority) by Catholics and Orthodox, and is considered apocryphal by Protestants, and does not carry much authority for many Jews (Armstrong, 2008). In the text, which was written in Greek as opposed to Hebrew, an angel gives instructions on catching and gutting a fish in order to burn parts for an exorcism to cure blindness (Tobit 6:8). This appears to be a form of folk medicine. The exorcism, which was an attempt to drive away the devil Asmodeus, would enshrine that particular demon into Western consciousness, as he was repeatedly attributed to be the possessing devil and was often associated with lust (Guiley, 2009).

In reviewing the sacred literature of the Mandeans (a small sect in Iraq with a very strong Jewish influence), Russell (2014) repeats the rite for a person possessed on a holy day. This involves mixing the saliva of a horse, the blood of both a pigeon and a monkey, adding mint and purslane to olive and sesame oil, and then placing this ointment in the possessed person's nose. Hoyt (1978) documents that later traditions included exorcisms assigned to characters from the Hebrew Scriptures. One such tradition identifies King Solomon as an exorcist, which is found in the *Testament of Solomon*, a Jewish text that dates to sometime between the 1st to 3rd century CE (Peterson, 1997).

Judging by the relative dearth of exorcism in the Hebrew Scriptures compared to the overwhelming frequency as cited in the Christian Scriptures, by the time of Jesus (roughly 4 BCE to 30 CE), exorcisms had become much more common among the Jewish community. This is further reinforced by what the Jewish historian Flavius Josephus (37-100 CE) reports in his text *Antiquities* (trans. 2001), which includes an exorcism performed by a Jewish man named Eleazer in front of the future Emperor Vespasian. In that exorcism, Eleazar invokes the name of Solomon to dispel the demon. The invocation of powerful names, including the use of the name of Jesus by those who were not specifically Christian, is cited in Mark 9:38 and appears to have the approval of the Gospel writer (Hoyt, 1978). Guiley (2009) notes that Josephus includes the widespread belief of the time that possession is often by those who had died at the hands of the conquering Romans. The early Christian saint Justin Martyr, writing around 150 CE, claims that possession was common among both Christians and Jews, as well as those who practiced more traditional polytheism practices common in the Greco-Roman world (Levack, 2013).

The Gospel of Mark has Jesus performing his first miracle as an exorcism (1:23-27). The demons throughout the Gospel stories are often connected with a form of physical illness (see Luke 7:21; Matthew 10:1). The three synaptic Gospels all include an incident when the exorcisms done by Jesus are questioned by the existing authorities, who claim that he must have that power from the devil. Guiley (2009) states that power over demons as a result of consorting with or having a pact with demons was a common belief in that era.

Ogden (2002), in his collection of primary sources from the classical world, posits that one reason for demonic possession and exorcisms increasing around the time of Jesus was that the Greek-speaking world connected hostile demons to murder or other violent death. The Roman (and the previous Greek) occupation of Israel resulted in multiple executions in order to maintain control (Crossan, 1999), thus a densely populated spiritual world of hostile demons that could torment the living was created. The classical poet Ovid (43 BCE-17/18 CE) claimed that the spirits of the dead would haunt the living, requiring a yearly ritual to exorcise their presence, going back to when Romulus the founder of Rome had killed his brother Remus (Hale, 2009). A related way of understanding this phenomenon is to view the persistent and ongoing generational trauma that the Jewish community faced with ongoing military occupation; coupled with the cognitive dissonance when this geopolitical reality was contrasted with the religiously held belief that YWHW had given the land of Israel to the Jewish people (see Joshua 21:43). This would give an added strength to one of the repeated possession-and-exorcism stories in the synoptic Gospels, that of the man possessed by multiple demons who identify themselves as "legion", which is a name for a division of Roman soldiers (Mark 5:9-10; Matthew 8:28-34; Luke 8:30).

It is understandable that this highly critical position of Rome as a demonic power becomes de-emphasized by the time the Gospels were written, as the conflict had escalated to the destruction of the Jewish Temple in CE 70, which is roughly when Mark was thought to be composed (Carroll, 2014). Russell (1977) argues that demonic understanding in Mark is focused on a specific figure of Satan. This is contrasted by the portrayal in Luke (which was composed later) where the power of the devil is seen in the authority of the religious institutional power structure. In the Gospel of John, the last of the canonical Gospels to be composed, Satan becomes fully connected to "the Jews" as a group. Within several centuries the Roman Empire itself becomes Christianized (Moss, 2013), but a sense of demonization of Jews clearly has continued to the present day, resulting in the nightmare of pogroms and the Holocaust, more accurately known as the *Shoah,* as that is the Hebrew word for catastrophe (Carroll, 2002; 2014).

Russell (1977) further advances the argument that it is a Hellenized Jewish world that changes the Jewish and emerging Christian thinking to include demons and exorcism. He notes that the possession stories, common in the Christian Scriptures, are usually lower demons, except in the Gospel of John, where it is always Satan. (One exception to this is Luke 22:3, when Satan possesses Judas before the betrayal of Jesus, see Bissell, 2016.) It is interesting to note that the Synoptic Gospels (Matthew, Mark and Luke), contain frequent exorcisms by Jesus; while John does not have a single exorcism (Hardy, 2014). Russell ascribes the evolution of thought about the devil to tension within Jewish monotheism; if God is all powerful (omnipotent) and all-good (omnibenevolent), then there must be a force for the evil in the world, which is either rebellious or subservient to God. As Russell puts it, “He is a counterpart, a doublet of the good Lord. He is the shadow of God” (Russell, 1977, p. 251).

There is one example within the Talmud (the Jewish religious commentary written about the Hebrew Scriptures after the destruction of the Jewish Temple in CE 70) that includes exorcism. Rabbi Simon orders an angel to possess the daughter of a king who is hostile to the Jewish diaspora (Kiely & McKenna, 2007). Note that this text has a lesser demon to do the “dirty work” of the Divine at the behest of the religious figure. Guiley (2009) notes that in succeeding centuries, Jewish belief in demons expanded and became a part of Kabbalistic lore in the Middle Ages.

The idea that the Jesus of history was possessed, or haunted, by God is one of the themes in Kazantzakis’ novel *The Last Temptation of Christ* (translated 1980), which was subsequently made into a movie of the same name by De Fina and Scorsese (1988). The very opening line of the novel states, “A cool heavenly breeze took possession of him” (Kazantzakis, 1980, p. 5). Davies (1995), in differentiating between spirit and demon possession, claims the main criterion is if the experience is beneficial to the group. Thus, in the Gospels, Mark 3:22-30 has the authorities questioning whether Jesus was possessed by an “unclean spirit”, i.e. a demon. For those within the Jesus movement (at least for Davies, 1995), Jesus was possessed by the Spirit of God in the same way that Borg (2001) noted the earlier Hebrew prophets were. However, for those who understood the Jesus movement as threatening, Jesus was demonic. It is worth noting, as Patterson (2014) does, that John the Baptist is also accused of being possessed by the crowd (Luke 7:33). Lewis (1986/2003) differentiates between central religions and peripheral cults. Using this criterion, the Jesus movement begins as a peripheral cult and moves to a central religion,

Christianity, eventually becoming the official religion of the Roman Empire.

As a bit of a tangential aside, Davies (1995) points out that while the move from peripheral cult to religion is probably most common, it is possible to go the other way as well. He gives the example of how Yoruba (including spirit possession) is a dominant religion in Nigeria, but becomes the peripheral possession cult of Santeria when practiced in Florida (see also Harrison, 2000; for a fictional portrayal of possession in Nigeria among the Ibo/Igbo people, see Achebe, 1958). Ward (1980), looking cross-culturally, and Shekar (1989), looking at possession in India, expand Lewis' (1986/2003) categories. For them, central religious spirit possession tends to be short-lived and never confused with illness. Peripheral possession, on the other hand, is seen by either the individual and/or their society as a form of illness needing treatment. However, the claim by Shekar (1989) that central religious possession is not connected with healing, while possibly true in India, seems to run contrary to Brown's (1991) claim that all Vodun (Voodoo) rituals are healing in some manner. While Vodun is a peripheral rite where Brown studied it in New York City, it is undoubtedly a central religion in Haiti and elsewhere (Harrison, 2000). Lloyd (2015b) cites a number of scholars who challenge Lewis' (1986/2003) dichotomy as being over simplistic and ignoring nuances in how cultures understand both spirits and various overlapping religious traditions.

Davies (1995) makes the argument that early Christianity arose from positive spirit possession as experienced by Jesus, his early followers, and St. Paul. This positive experience of possession was coupled with the healing that occurred when those who had negative experiences of spirit possession (i.e. demonic possession) were cured. Patterson (2014) identifies those negative possession experiences as struggles with what would now be called mental health issues, although I find that reading a little narrow (although it seems certain that mental health struggles then, and for some now, can be understood as demonic). For Davies (1995), and Lampe (1972) before him, the theory that Jesus experienced the "spirit of God" as a form of possession-trance solves a divide that splits the world of historical Jesus scholarship. For many Jesus scholars of the more liberal inclinations, Jesus did not claim divine status (e.g. Borg, 1995, 2001; Crossan, 1999; Spong, 1995) but was given that position after his death by subsequent generations. For orthodox Christians, statements of the divinity of Jesus are a part of the faith (Nolan, 1989). Davies overcomes this divide by allowing the historical Jesus to have purely human attributes, and another persona to be the "spirit of God". It is worth noting, as documented by Ehrman (2014), that this belief in the human Jesus possessed by the Spirit of God (or at least adopted by the Divine) had an ancient heritage but was later deemed heretical and labeled Theodotianism after the founder of the thought, Theodotus. Ehrman (2014) points out that this belief has at least some traces that go back to the earliest days of Christianity.

After the death and resurrection of Jesus, the canonical book *The Acts of the Apostles* documents a form of positive possession occurring on the Jewish feast of Pentecost among those remaining members of Jesus' inner circle (Acts Chapter 2), an event sometimes marked as the birthdate of Christianity. Those who were gathered heard a rushing wind, saw flames over their heads, and were able to speak in tongues, utilizing languages they did not know in order to speak to those who were gathered for the feast. (It is also possible this was glossolalia and was not a specific language.) Crabtree (1997a) places this event within the context of Jewish apocalyptic expectation, with an oppressed and occupied society on edge and hopeful for divine intervention against the power of Rome (see also Carroll, 2014). As the Christian movement aged into the second generation, the dynamism of spirit possession moved into spirit inspiration, a pattern that can be seen in other religious movements like the Society of Friends, also known as Quakers (Dandelion, 2008) and more contemporarily in Pentecostalism (Cuneo, 2001).

Possession in the early to Medieval Christian Church

Demos (2008) notes how early Christian communities in places throughout the Roman Empire experienced significant suspicion by both neighbors and authorities. Some of this is due to misunderstanding the rituals and practices of the early Church. A community that engaged in radical equality and greeted each other with a kiss of peace became, among detractors, a community engaging in incest like the mythic Oedipus. Communal gatherings that included Eucharistic meals involving consuming what was said to be the blood and flesh of their human God became known as Thyestean Feasts, or cannibalism. The rejection of aspects of the Imperial Religion, in which most Christians refused to participate in the worship of the Emperor, led to charges of heresy, atheism, and black magic. In 177 CE in what is now Lyons, France, rumors of cannibalistic rituals by incestuous Christians (who were supposedly particular to the flesh of newborn children) led the local authorities to begin a criminal investigation that eventually led to executions (or in Christian understanding, martyrdom). Incest, heresy, murder and cannibalism are all charges that will be repeated throughout history against the communities of those perceived to be "Others" in order to enforce conformity.

It is not to be assumed that Roman authority was alone in demonizing their opponents. There is a long history within the Christian tradition of connecting pagan worship to demonic activity. Bissell (2016) notes in Paul's First Letter to the Corinthians a prohibition from too close a connection with non-Jewish (pagan) butchers, as invariably the animal was involved in some form of ritual sacrifice. 1 Corinthians 10:20-21 states, "No, but the sacrifices of pagans are offered to demons, not to God, and I do not want you to be participants with demons. You cannot drink the cup of the Lord and the cup of demons too; you cannot have a part in both the Lord's table and the table of demons." Bissell (2016) then notes that Paul backtracks, as when a Christian is invited to share a meal with a pagan, one should eat whatever is set before you (10:27). Bissell notes that "Paul, for his gifts, must have been a triumphantly confusing teacher" (p. 66*n*).

One of the early followers of Christianity was Matthew, who is also the supposed author of one of the Gospels. Bissell (2016) points out a tradition mentioned in the writings of Clement of Alexandria (115-215 CE) that Matthew was a vegetarian, which would possibly connect him to Jewish Christian practices centered around James, the brother of Jesus, at least until the Temple was destroyed in 70 CE. In praising Matthew's diet, "…Clement believed that the 'most suitable' foods were those 'fit for immediate use without fire' and argued that an overreliance on cooked meat could lead to a 'Belly-demon', which in Clement's mind was 'the worst and most abandoned of demons'" (p. 336). This approach runs counter to some contemporary Christian opposition to vegetarianism (see page 88) but also has similarities to the raw food movement of today.

The Franciscan priest Richard Rohr (2007) makes a direct connection between Biblical understandings of demonic possession and contemporary understandings of addiction. For Rohr, the treatment of addiction, like exorcism, must be done in a social context and be motivated by compassion. However, he does not explore this idea further. In the early Christian church, converts (catechumens) underwent an 8-week process of "daily instructions, austerities, healings and exorcisms" (Brock & Parker, 2008, p. 122). Explaining the process, Brock and Parker (2008) state that the exorcisms freed the new converts from the control of outside influences. These could include not just compulsions, but also antisocial behavior, physical illness, and even oppressive government. Such beliefs in the power of spiritual forces seem common in the ancient world, with a few exceptions. One cited is Lucian of Samosata (120-192 CE), a satirist who seems to be one of the few of his contemporaries who ridiculed exorcisms. For him, belief in spirit possessions was due to corruptions from outside of the civilized, Greek-speaking world, an observation that runs counter to Ogden's (2002) research.

Theology around baptism reflects the importance of exorcism in the thought of the early church (Baglio, 2009; Brock & Parker, 2008). For the early Christian teacher St. John Chrysostom (CE 349-407), possession can purify a person for heaven (Stevenson, 2007). This theme, while not common, does continue to have resonance as several saints were supposed to be possessed, including St. John Vianney (1786-1859) for the whole of his life. Vianney was also known for his skills in exorcism, although he never appeared to get around to performing an exorcism on Antoine Gay (1790-1871), who is reported to have remained possessed for the rest of his life, eventually dying as a Third Order Franciscan who scourged himself and lived on a diet of bread and water (Phillips, 2015c). The Belgium folk saint Christina the Astonishing (1150-1224) was incarcerated at least twice due to her odd and erratic behavior, such as burning and freezing herself as well as levitating (Young, 2018). Her behavior was initially attributed to possession but later in her life it was assumed to be a sign of her holiness. There are signs of her having epilepsy and possibly serious mental health concerns such as Borderline Personality Disorder (Kelly & Rogers, 1993). Marie Des Valles (1590-1656) reported that she was possessed for 30 years after spurning the attentions of a suitor, and engaged in very public acts of penance, including circling churches on her knees as she could not enter them (Werse, 2015a). A more modern and less obscure example would be Mother Theresa of Calcutta (1910-1997), who underwent an exorcism toward the end of her life and famously had dealt with a dark night of the soul for many years (Phillips, 2015b).

It should be noted that in the early Church baptism was almost exclusively for adults, sometimes near their death, as in the case of the Emperor Constantine (CE 272-327). Before baptism the catechumen would *Exsufflatio* (literally "out breathing") by rejecting the devil and *Insufflatio* (literally "in-breathing") by inhaling the breath of the priest (Phillips, 2015a). Schull (2015) claims that this rite created a clear break from the pre-conversion life of the catechumen. Of course, for some that was the reason to postpone the baptism, so one did not need to make significant life changes until they were much older when it was (presumably) easier to be good. An advantage to the public exorcisms that Brock and Parker (2008) studied is that, instead of the isolated and atomized tendency of Western healing (including psychotherapy), these public exorcisms dealt with the complex and relational realities of the lived experience of catechumens.

In the earliest days of Christianity, exorcisms could be performed by anyone. As the Church aged, more formal understandings quickly became apparent, often leading to conflicts (see Ehrman, 2005). Pope Cornelius wrote a letter to the Bishop of Antioch in 253 CE which mentions the city of Rome having 52 official exorcists. Kiely & McKenna (2007) note that Rome had approximately 30,000 believers at that time, meaning one exorcist was available to every 577 Christians. The Council of Laodicea (363) banned those not invested by a bishop from performing an exorcism (Baglio, 2009).

Kathleen Norris is an author best known for her creative, spiritual nonfiction (1997, 2001). In her most recent work in that genre, *Acedia & Me* (2008), she critiques the existing psychological establishment for missing the spiritual dimension in life. Her writing style weaves personal experience, in this case, her husband's long struggles with physical and mental illness until his eventual death, and exegesis of ancient texts. *Acedia & Me* focuses on the fourth-century desert monk Evagruis Ponticus (for more on Ponticus, see also Bamberger, 2006). Norris says that what we label as "an individual's issues" would have been called, in the desert monastic tradition, "demons" (2008). Evagruis' insights into the human condition include his observations that moods and thoughts are directly connected to specific locations in the brain, an observation only recently discovered by neuropsychology (Bamberger, 2006). The desert monks, while focused on demons, did not concern themselves with exorcisms. For them, as the monastic scholar Crislip (2005) notes, demons led to temptations that often were only thoughts (after all, they had removed many if not most physical temptations by moving to the deserts). Wilson-Hartgrove (2008) writes about how St. Anthony (251-356 CE), one of the key figures of the desert monastic tradition and a famous demon battler, stood for both personal as well as social transformation. It is noted that the battles with the devil are not just psychological or spiritual conflicts that are internal, they are also about the dominant culture of the Roman Empire (albeit a newly Christian Empire) and a more radical understanding of the call of religion. The image of Anthony battling demons in the desert would remain a common theme throughout the Middle Ages (Wilkinson, 2015) and it is believed that Anthony's experiences as an exorcist helped inform the early Church (Guiley, 2009). John Cassian (CE 360-433) promoted the belief that demons had specialties in the temptations toward sin, such as the demon of anger (Cassian & Gibson, 2018).

Many saints are reported to have engaged in exorcisms, to the point where Kallendorf (2003) argues that many saintly biographies include exorcisms as a part of the hagiography genre. For example, while Salzmann (2015) claims that St. Augustine of Hippo (354-430) performed exorcisms which were as graphic as any in a contemporary film. Kallendorf (2003) claims those are later stories not found in the saint's own voluminous works. Peters (2004) writes about Pope Gregory I (540-604), often referred to as "The Great" due to the numerous reforms he instituted throughout the Western Church as well as his extensive writings, which include 850 letters. Gregory's reforms led to a creative and more organized monasticism, whose influence on Western Monasticism shaped society throughout the Middle Ages. One story of the miracle-working Pope, as cited by Hoyt (1978), includes the successful exorcism of a young girl by a bishop after the failure of exorcism by a local female "witch". Peters (2004) writes,

> Sixth century Christianity demonstrated a heightened interest in demons, miracles and holy men and women. Although Gregory could not do away with this new fascination, his stories could at least show that demons were always defeated by simple Christian practices. Demons and sorcerers were a vivid part of Gregory's universe, but they were kept firmly under control by none other than simple Christian practices and demonstrations of sanctity. (p. 130)

Scull (2015) argues that exorcisms, especially among those who were pagan in Northern Europe, were a key part of Christian evangelization of the time.

The figure of Benedict of Nursia (480-543 CE) was a highly influential person in the Western Christian tradition, in large part because his monastic rule became the primary organizational model for monastics and increasingly "secular" clergy (Cook, 2009). Tradition has it that he had exorcised demons from the location of the Benedictine home monastery, Monte Cassino, as well as used exorcism prayers to protect himself from a poisoning by disgruntled monks (Hoyt, 1978). It should be noted that these stories are not included in the biography of him as written by Gregory, but appear to be a later tradition (Knight, 2012). However, this tradition has led to the widespread use of a medal with Benedict's image upon it, used by Catholics since at least 1664 (Blosser, 2015). It is sometimes referred to as the "exorcist medal", although it was worn by lay and clergy alike and the prayers associated with it could be said by any baptized person. There are several variations of the shape and the writing on the medal, but all have Benedict, a cross, and various Latin letters. One variation, V.R.S.N.S.M.V.–S.M.Q.L.I.V.B., began to be used in 1647 when several Bavarian witches claimed they could not practice magic near a Benedictine monastery that had in its possession a cross with those letters on it, although no one knew what they meant. Wisely, someone searched the library to discover a 15th century text including an exorcism that was, in Latin: "*Vade retro Satana*! *Nunquam suade mihi vana*! *Sunt mala quae libas. Ipse venena bibas*!"

("Begone, Satan! Never tempt me with your varieties! What you offer me is evil. Drink the poison yourself!" Blosser, 2015, p. 38).

Demos (2008) notes a cultural change in the early medieval period. During the reign of Charlemagne, roughly 768-814, sorcery was condemned but so was accusing others of witchcraft, a crime which could be punished by death, presumably due to the widespread pre-Christian practices still in effect. By the 10th century, pagan practices appear to have continued, however they were now more severely punished, and there was no longer a prohibition of accusing a person of witchcraft. The possessed person, by the late 7th century in Europe, like a witch, was often a woman (Russell, 1972). There is widespread near scholarly consensus that much of this phenomenon in Europe is, at least in part, due to the continuation of pre-Christian practices throughout Europe during the Middle Ages (Cook, 2009). The Christian conversion process was not without conflict; Pye (2014) wryly tells of St. Willibrord (658-739), who was struck by the guardian of an idol after the saint had defaced the idol. Of course, in the hagiography it is the guardian who is seen as possessed and yet is saved from the threatening crowd by the injured saint. The guardian still died three days later, "as persons who have been seized by crowds tend to do" (p. 8).

It is worth remembering that the process of Christianization outside the urban areas of the former Roman Empire took centuries, as an outlier it was not completed in Lithuania until the 14th century CE (Peters, 2004). Even then, folk practices were retained for centuries in many parts of Europe. Pagan folk practices did not die out easily. Hoyt (1978) tells some of the story of James Murrell (1785-1860), one of the last Cunning Men of England (also known as folk magicians or white wizards, although Mr. Murrell's death certificate lists him as a "quack doctor"). Murrell was available to cast spells and conjure missing items, and did engage in exorcisms, usually by placing iron jars containing something of the possessed person into a fire. The bottles would inevitably explode, thereby healing the ill or possessed person, although readers are left to wonder if any were injured by shrapnel.

Bernard of Clairvaux (1090-1153) was a hugely influential churchman for good and for bad, writing influentially and beautifully on numerous spiritual subjects, working on monastic reforms and unfortunately encouraging the 2nd Crusade (Cook, 2009). Numerous exorcisms by the saint are recorded, including a humorous dialogue reproduced by Hoyt (1978):

> A crowd had gathered to witness the battle between the saint and the devil. Immediately the devil spoke up, taunting the saint. 'No', said the devil, 'this eater of leeks, this devourer of cabbages shall not drive me away'. ...He

> fastened a sign around her neck and the devil never came to her again. (pp. 21-22)

Bredero (2001) includes the posthumous use of Bernard's beard hairs by a confrere in literally chasing a devil.

While Christian history and Islamic history both tend to be viewed in isolation, without a doubt they had a clear pull upon each other. This was due to territory being quickly conquered by Islamic armies, starting in the 7th century CE. The Quran has little about health and disease, so pre-Islamic animistic traditions that attributed many diseases to the influence of jinn had a significant influence on Islamic thought then and into the present day (Scull, 2015). Muhammad is not recorded as engaging in healings or exorcisms in the Quran, although these stories do appear later in the tradition among the *Haditha*, or stories about the Prophet (Scull, 2015).

Western Europe began a significant cultural transformation around the year 1000 CE, in part due to the interaction with more advanced Islamic civilization (Peters, 2004). There was an increase in literary and philosophical output, including the new scholastic methods that included inter-textual debate, such as Thomas Aquinas' question "if Christians can seek the aid of demons" (as cited in Peters, 2004, p. 333). Rubenstein (2003) notes that the popularity of Aristotle was a significant factor in this change, as much of his work, as well as Islamic commentary on his work, became available in Latin only at this time. Unlike his fellow Classical philosophers like Plato (known in the Middle Ages as "The Philosopher"), Aristotle questioned the existence of demons. That aspect of his philosophy did not gain widespread acceptance at this time, however. Kugel (2011) notes that also at this time the use of trial by ordeal (such as having an accused person hold onto a red-hot piece of metal to determine guilt) decreased, due in part to the acceptance of a more naturalistic explanation for the world. Scull (2015) notes how, in parallel, during the 12th century CE in China, the attribution of illness to demonic forces decreased, especially among the elite. Instead, healers looked to internal imbalances, such as the lack of *qi*. It does appear that the use of exorcism was still widely practiced in China at this time, however, as the elite was a very small group, consisting of perhaps 1-2% of the population.

Between the 1300s and the 1600s, fear of the power of supernatural forces reached a height in Europe, as seen in witch trials and many exorcisms, both often focused on women. One example of collective fear was the Spanish Inquisition. Originally designed to detect non-devout members of those who had converted to Christianity from Islam or Judaism as a part of the *Reconquista* that occurred on the Iberian Peninsula (Cook, 2009), the Inquisition helped shape the notion of an ethnic identity to the modern nation state (Carroll, 2009). Hoyt (1978) cites a Spanish Jesuit tract of that time that included exorcisms designed to drive demons from a specific location. Scull (2015) argues that the popularity of morality plays, which could be performed by traveling troupes or were connected to a particular location at a specific time, encouraged possession narratives, although no citation is offered for this theory.

Throughout most of recorded history, Taylor notes (2007), beating a possessed person was considered proper treatment in order to make the demon uncomfortable, a position that Hardtke (2015) claimed was made almost institutional by John Duns Scotus (1266-1308). For example, St. Norbert of Magdeburg (1080-1134) had a possessed woman plunged into water after having her head shaved (Hoyt, 1978). Similar approaches were taken for suspected witches and those who were thought to be to changelings, that is, children believed to have been switched by fairies or other preternatural beings (Butler, 2015). Martin Luther was said to have exorcised a young girl with a strong stick (Hardtke, 2015) and further suggested a young boy who did nothing but eat and defecate be suffocated after suspecting he was sired by the devil; the townspeople refused to harm or exorcise the child but he died within a year (Miles, 2005). Even as recent as 1895, an Irish woman was tortured and burned alive by her husband and other family members due to the fact that they believed she was a changeling and that the "real" woman would be returned by the fairies (Butler, 2015).

Pye (2014) notes that at times, those who were seen as mad or possessed could be protected; this was the case with the vicar Hugh of St. Martin who, in 1298, went mad and pawned all his clothes. Those who injured him were excommunicated. Also, a clerk who killed his master while possessed in 1285 was pardoned due to his impairment (Pye, 2014). The shrine of St. Dymphna in Gheel, located in modern-day Belgium, was a location for those who were struggling with madness and included areas to chain the afflicted, so they could undergo the 18 days of exorcism. However, if the person was not cured, they were allowed to move into the surrounding community (Scull, 2015).

Johnson (2008), building upon the work of Lewis (1986/2003), notes that medieval women were also able to use positive possession in the form of visions of the divine in order to comment upon and critique existing power. Women who did so successfully include St. Bridget of Sweden (1303-1373), who made general commentaries about the state of the church. St. Catherine of Siena (1347-1380) famously criticized the Papacy after the move from Rome to Avignon. Such commentary would be unlikely without the protection offered through the women's visionary experience. The Beguine community was a semi-monastic lay movement that was outside hierarchal control. One member, Marie d'Oignies (1177-1213), was said to have the power of exorcism, although she appeared to be careful to defer to male advice about what to do regarding demons, which may be why she became formally recognized as blessed by the Catholic Church and was not tried as a heretic (Pye, 2014).

In a review of thirteenth-century hagiographies (a formulaic genre of saintly biographies), Espí Forcén and Espí Forcén (2014) note the recurring thematic trope of demonic possession and attribute it in part to the workings of the genre, but also accede to a familiarity in the lived experiences of the (mostly anonymous) authors. Wilkinson (2007) notes that the power of the devil is an explanation for the suffering, illnesses, and pain of a hard life. The influences of devils (and witches) were not the only medical theory that existed for the ancients. Hoyersten (1996) notes the prevalence of astrological understandings, as well as the theory of bodily humors, which goes back to the classical medical understanding of the Greek doctor practicing in Rome Galen (130-210 CE), and the Hippocratic tradition he worked within. This was an approach that was distinct from priestly and folk healing traditions common in the ancient world (Scull, 2015). Moses (2009) tells of how Francis of Assisi (1181-1226) viewed warfare in the neighboring town of Arezzo as of demonic origin and ordered his confrere, Brother Sylvester, to exorcise the devils at the city gate. It is worthy to note that Francis himself was unable to be present, which is unexplained in the original documents but which Moses (2009) attributes to Francis' own PTSD symptoms after his struggles on the battlefield and subsequently as a prisoner of war.

Spirit Possession in Asia

The sub-continent of India and the ancient religious traditions of Hinduism have already been addressed several times throughout this text. Tantric practices in Hinduism and Buddhism include a tradition of possession going back to at least the 8th century CE (Elby, 2015a). Both positive possession by a deity or the deceased soul of a guru, and negative possession by a malevolent deity appear to be considered possibilities within the traditions. Specifically, Shaivistic tantra is characterized by a worship of Shiva and views demonic possession as dealing with lesser emanations of the Divine. Devotees may seek out possession as a goal in a progressive spiritual path. Practitioners often sought out "impure" locations such as cremation grounds. Later thinkers such as Abhinavagupta (950-1016 CE) tended to domesticate these approaches by emphasizing visualization of the acts as opposed to engaging in them physically. This makes this approach seem similar to tantra practices in Tibet (Elby, 2015a). In the Indian state of Kerala, *teyyam* practices are common, where either Hindu priests devoted to a specific deity or professional performers become voluntarily possessed by any of the Hindu pantheon (Elby, 2015b). The dances are highly stylized and include elaborate costuming.

Given that a central tenet of Buddhism is the illusionary nature of the personality, possession can be understood somewhat differently than in other philosophies (Padoan, 2015). Buddhism was especially open to the integration of indigenous religious practices, including native gods. They were seen as either protectors of the Dharma (literally, the Law) or as ignorant entities in need of enlightenment. Both types of spiritual beings were capable of possessing a person, including monks as well as laypeople. Varieties of possession are well documented in areas as diverse as Tibet (which has a strong Tantric influence) and Sri Lanka. That country's Galle area is known for a ritual dance with a male exorcist who cross-dresses as a female to lure a cemetery dwelling demon into a cock. Burmese Buddhist practices also include cross-dressing mediums who are spiritually married to one of the 37 possible deities known as *nats* (Perriere & Rozenberg, 2015). That form of possession begins unintentionally and often includes mental health and physical complaints until the underlying reason is discovered by a more experienced medium. In Mongolia, among the Darhad people, the personality is understood to be balanced between a Buddhist yellow side and a shamanistic black side. Possession allows that black side to be manifest (Padoan, 2015). Thailand's northeastern villages will have both Buddhist monks (who tend to the men for healing) and shamans, many of whom are illiterate and relegated to treating female health and spiritual needs.

Tibetan Buddhism has a unique form of ritualized exorcism known as "chod", which is a shortening of the longer Tibetan "*dud kyi chod yul*" or "severance of the demonic object" (McNamara, 2015). In general, the practice is a series of progressive visualizations that can be accompanied by music, including the performance of a trumpet made from a human femur. The person engaging in the ritual may do it in a frightening or disturbing location. The visualizations include: cutting open the head to allow the consciousness of the world to enter, then dismembering the body and placing it in the empty skull to feed the world, thus leading to the eradication of demons. Four levels of demons are understood to be affected by the practice; material demons (who are out to hurt the practitioner); immaterial demons (such as a practitioner's own doubts and fears); exaltation demons (an inflated sense of a practitioner's spiritual progress); and the inflation demon (the rejection of the inherent suffering in all life).

Tibet has also had a long history of oracles, some of whom, like the *Nechung*, are believed to have been evil spirits once exorcised and now serving for the benefit of the community. The *Nechung* holds an almost official role as an advisor to the Dalai Lama (Bell, 2015a). Tibetan exorcisms can include offering barley dough formed into a crude human form; these can include hair and/or nail clippings of the possessed person in an effort to draw out the spirit (Bell, 2015b). Welwood (2000) notes that Tibetan Buddhist practice incorporates shamanistic and magical actions, stemming from the acceptance of native beliefs when Buddhism was introduced to the country in the 8th century CE.

Japan has experienced a long history of belief in possession states (Hoyt, 1978), including a variety of different expressions throughout history and into the modern day (Dolce, 2015). Shinto, the traditional indigenous religion with roots that include shamanism, has a trance dance known as *kagura* that is the probable origin for the better-known *Noh* theatre, which notably includes masked figures (Mikles, 2015a). Shinto also had a long history of *miko* mediums, females who become possessed by indigenous deities who can tell fortunes, exorcise unwanted spirits, and ritually bless visitors to the shrine. Mikles (2015b) notes how *miko* were suppressed with the strengthening of Japanese central rule in the 7th century CE. However, they have a continued presence in Shinto rituals in the role of assistants. In the present day, they are seen primarily in rural Japan.

Other Japanese possession states include various Buddhist practices, such as the rites of *Abisha*, when a spirit (usually identified as a fox), is brought out of the possessed person by the ritual chanting of a Buddhist priest and sent into a third person. The third person is often either a child or a young woman, although sometimes even noble ladies played such a role (Blacker, 1975). In these cases, the newly possessed person usually would scream and throw themselves onto the ground, although the literature suggests that the state seems to pass quickly. These rituals seem especially common among followers of the Nichiren teachings of Japanese Buddhism (Hoyt, 1978), which emphasized ritual chanting, especially of certain sutras (Matthews, 1995). Sometimes a meal would be prepared for the departing spirit, or the possessed person would be threatened in the hope that the fox spirit would leave (Hoyt, 1978). The fox as a character appears in Murakami's novel *The Wind-Up Bird Chronicles* (1994) along with more modern deities, including Col. Sanders from Kentucky Fried Chicken. This form of Buddhism is seen to be in contrast to the more widely known Zen form, with an emphasis upon meditation (Matthews, 1995).

Hoyt (1978) reports on European Catholic missionaries in Japan who, in 1565, attempted exorcisms on a family that claimed 100 years of possession. It is not examined in the text how the Christian approach would have differed from contemporary Japanese practices, and soon after Japan closed itself to outsiders, including Western missionaries (Cook, 2009). In Japan, members of so-called "new religions" (as opposed to the old religions of Shinto and Buddhism, and foreign religions such as Christianity), often complain of possession by spirits of people or animals (Goodman, 1988b). One of the main activities of these religions is healing those who are physically, mentally, or spiritually ill. One of these religions, Tenrikyo, was founded by Nakayama Miki (1798-1887), a peasant woman who experienced possession by *Tenri O no Mikoto*, who claimed to be the Creator Spirit. There was the clear influence of earlier Nichiren Buddhism practices upon this tradition. Miki's revelations lasted 50 years and are recorded in 3 books sacred to the tradition (Hardy, 2014).

These New Religions have had negative press, such as the execution of Sachita Eto in 2012 for 6 deaths in one year due to his use of beating sticks during exorcisms. It has been argued by Murguia (2015) that these spiritual expressions became common due in part to the suppression of more traditional Shinto practices after Japan's defeat in World War II. A number of current religious leaders are cited as examples of messianic and charismatic leaders who claim possession by deities and/or historic persons. One such figure is Ryuho Okawa (b. 1956), who has channeled various persons ranging from the guardian angel of Kim Jong Il and Zeus, as well as Isaac Newton. Okawa maintains a Facebook presence under the name Happy Science.

Exorcism practices in Malaysia include a ritual where an exorcist has spirits enter jars of water and then, as the spirits are often in the form of ferocious animals, engages in a type of battle with them to drive them away (Hoyt, 1978). Hoyt (1978) further notes that possession by animal spirits is common in China as well. These spirits were specifically cited in the work of a Presbyterian missionary John L. Nevius (1829-1893), who attempted to change some approaches of foreign missions, including building churches in the local style. Far from being a complete syncretist, Nevius also condemned existing Chinese practices as demonic. Nevius built upon existing animistic beliefs and wrote a text on his exorcism work, as well as that of his Chinese Christian converts (Nevius, 1894). One of the advantages the mission appeared to have was the apparent successes over traditional healers in exorcising spirits (Hoyt, 1978) as well as the convert's fearlessness in staying in supposed haunted houses (Nevius, 1894). It is interesting that Nevius found the possession state to be common but that post-exorcism, those once possessed were loath to discuss the situation, attributing a degree of shame to the experience.

There is a well-documented rejection or downplaying of this possession tradition throughout Chinese history, going back to Doaist writers around 300 CE (Haar, 2015). While Doaism places a strong emphasis on spirit possession as a cause of much of human suffering, it is believed that exorcism ought to be an extreme last resort, with more emphasis being placed upon proper diet, proper behavior, and seeking spiritual guidance as effective remedies (Greer, 2015). This clearly differs from cultures that prefer spirit possession and subsequent exorcism to other explanations of suffering (see Baglio, 2009, for Italy as an example of such a culture).

Korea has a long history of shamanistic practices stretching to long before the arrival of Buddhism, usually by women (Wood, 2015a). At present, there are two different types of shamans in Korea, *tanggol* and *mudang*. *Tanggol* inherit their position from the previous generation, are found around the southern coast, and do not exhibit possession in their rituals, which are more in line with the existing Buddhist and Christian practices of much of the population. *Mudang* shamans, on the other hand, are found around Seoul and areas north, are "called" to their practice after experiencing hardships such as abuse or depression, and must be initiated into the work. The social status of the shaman is very low within South Korea and s/he is persecuted in North Korea (which, as a Communist country, is officially atheistic); although in both countries it appears that many continue to visit shamans, including professional persons.

Birtalan (2015) notes how the Mongolian people of modern-day Mongolia, China, and Russia have a blended religious system that has retained their long-held shamanistic practices as well as integrating influences from Uigur Islam and Tibetan Buddhism. The Mongolian language has several words to differentiate ranks and types of shamans, as well as others who enter trance states, such as bards who recite long epic poems that can be modified to include specific ritual needs of the community. Vietnam has 54 different ethnic groups and a variety of religious influences, including not only Buddhism and Catholicism but also the Mother Goddess Religion known as Đạo Mãu, which explicitly includes possession by benevolent deities, and Trãn Hu'ng Đạo, a religion that worships a 13th century general who defended the country from Mongol invaders. Followers of that religion will cut their tongues in order to bleed on paper, the patterns of which are interpreted for messages.

Spirit Possession in Islam

In a research study done with Bangladeshi immigrants in London, Dien, Alexander and Napier (2008) document through snowball interviews (one interviewee suggests the next interviewee) that most exorcisms done in the community consist of a repetition of Koranic verses and/or traditional Islamic prayers over water, which is then drunk. Dein and Samad Illaiee (2009) document how olive oil is also often ingested as a part of Islamic exorcisms, which might involve a week or so of prayers and water and/or oil consumption. Throughout Islamic practice, the recitation of Quranic verses is a key part of the community's sacred activity (Eneborg, 2015).

Aslam (2015) notes how common belief in possession and jinn exists throughout Pakistan, although there are some fundamentalist Muslims who deny that possibility due to the lack of information in the Quran. Many of the openings for possession in that culture are directly tied to social mores, for example unbraided hair for women is supposedly a trap for spirits. Possamai (2015) notes a tension within the European Muslim community between Salafi interpretations, which tend to be more legalistic and orthodox, and *marabouts*, a type of folk healer found in traditional communities in Northern and Western Africa who use amulets and increasingly advertise online, on TV, and on the radio (see also Labous, 2015). The Salafi Muslim community has their own exorcists known as *raqis* (Possamai, 2015).

Mass Hysteria

There is evidence that possession is possibly contagious. Numerous anthropological studies report cases of group possession (Goodman, 1988b; Herskovits, 1971; Huxley, 1971; Winzeler, 2012). Carl Jung (1968) in fact combines the phenomenon of possession with mass hysteria, a description that is overly broad but does contain a degree of observational accuracy. Beginning in 1318 and continuing through to the sixteenth century, outbreaks of ecstatic dance swept over Western Europe, known either as St. John's, St. Vitus', or Tarantella Dance (Russell, 1972), although clinically it is known as imitative chorea (Laycock, 2015b). The association of St. Vitus is due to an occasion in Strasbourg, France, when the dancers were taken to the chapel of the saint to be prayed over and have the demons exorcised (Hoyt, 1978). St. John's became associated due to the period of time when the dancing outbreaks were common, given that they occurred near the Summer Solstice, on the Feast of St. John the Baptist (Laycock, 2015b). It should be noted that Tarantella Dance is a related but different phenomenon; the tarantella is a spider (wolf spider) and from the 11th to the 17th century in Italy it was believed that those who were bitten must dance to not succumb to the effects of the venom; those who were once bitten had to return yearly to local chapels or churches where music would be played (Laycock, 2015b). Dancers would continue to dance until exhausted, falling over themselves and often calling out the names of demons. Generally, they were poor and the majority appear to have been women (Russell, 1972), a similar population to those who had experienced possession states.

A historical understanding of this phenomenon must include the effects of plague as well as famine, which led to major movements of populations in a time that discouraged social change, understandably causing a great deal of individual anxiety and trauma (Russell, 1972). Demos (2008) states that the Black Death, beginning in 1350, and the Hundred Years War between France and England, were two enormously disrupting events within Western Europe. Demos (2008) notes that while individual accusations of witchcraft were common in small villages and hamlets, witch panics tended to be centered in larger communities where people were not all known to each other.

Koning (2013) attributes an inherent human tendency toward envy and deceit manifesting with significant agricultural changes as a part of the historical outbreak of possession narratives then and now, as this appears to be a dynamic currently being played out in sub-Saharan Africa, which makes a degree of sense given there have been no comparable group possession outbreaks in Europe since the late 19th century (Levack, 2013). Peters (2004) points to long stretches of famine in Europe, especially from 1309 to 1314 CE. This was in addition to poor knowledge of nutritional needs among all sections of society and diets that were poor in basic staples such as fruits and vegetables in the long winter. In speaking of the effects of poor nutrition, Peters states, "The psychological consequences include depression and despair, increasing hatred of aliens and the prosperous groups, and widespread complaints about dysfunctional social institutions, including social disorder and violence" (2004, p. 363). This environment appears to set the stage for mass possessions as well as fear of the power of outside forces, including spiritual ones, upon the collective.

There have been some, such as Caporeal (1976), who attempt to connect witch crazes and other forms of mass hysteria to outbreaks of ergot. Ergot is a mold that grows on grain, especially rye, and can cause hallucinations and convulsions in people with vitamin A deficiencies (Laycock, 2015c). While there are clear similarities between ergotism, possession states, and dancing hysteria, Laycock (2015c) cautions against any easy explanations when examining historic phenomena such as mass hysteria.

Possession and subsequent exorcisms and witch hysteria tend to occur in clusters or waves (Midelfort, 2005). Guiley (2009) reports on several Ursuline nuns in a convent located in Aix-en-Provence who experienced possession after at least one had an affair with her confessor priest. The possessions, which lasted from 1609-1611, ended with the torture and execution of the priest and a visually impaired village girl being accused of assisting the priest. One of the religious sisters, Madeleine de Demandolx de la Palud, was accused of witchcraft later in her life.

Aldous Huxley's book *The Devils of Loudan* (1971) chronicles a case of hysteria within a convent in France from 1617-1634. In that situation, the nuns claimed bewitchment from Fr. Urbain Grandier, a handsome priest notorious for his infidelities. Initially the mother superior was the only one possessed. She had several physical challenges and is reported to have had a difficult personality. Quickly more of the sisters exhibited signs of possession until Fr. Grandier was arrested, accused of heresy and witchcraft, and burned at the stake in 1634. However, possession of some of the sisters and subsequent exorcisms continued until 1660. Huxley (1971) ended the novel with the line, "The long orgy was at an end. If there had been no exorcists, it would never have begun" (quoted in Hoyt, 1978, p. 39). The argument that exorcism leads to people being labeled possessed, thus needing an exorcism, is echoed by Levacek (2013) in looking at celebrity exorcists like the contemporaries Frs. Fortea and Amroth as well as historic exorcists like Glassner. Huxley's book was later made into a movie titled *The Devils* (Baird, Russell & Solo, 1971), although the historically unattractive mother superior was played by the very attractive Vanessa Redgrave.

In writing about the incident, Werse (2015c) notes several theories as to what was occurring. This includes the rise of female focused spirituality at the time, which resulted in an increase in the ability for the nuns to be heard. Thus, their possession states were a form of protest to the sexual exploitation inflicted upon them by their chaplain. Possamai (2015) notes how the crowds that were in attendance for the exorcisms and later trials helped to strengthen social and cultural ties. Guiley (2009) noted some idiosyncratic traits that came out in the trial of Fr. Grandier, including his contact with the demon Ashtraoth that was limited to between 10 and 11 pm on Wednesdays.

France was also the location of a large witch craze from 1627 to 1630 in Mattaincourt, which included Fr. Dominic Gordet. Gordet was convicted of seducing several women who were being tried for witchcraft, although it seems likely he had sexual relations with more than those he admitted to. His entire testimony, though, is somewhat suspect as it was provided while under torture (Monter, 2015). In general, France had fewer episodes of possession and/or witch hysteria, which Demos (2008) claims was due to the relative strength of the central State.

Johann Weyer (1515-1588) attributed the symptoms often viewed as related to witchcraft to mental illness after witnessing an outbreak of mass hysteria in 1545 (Cumo, 2015b). Weyer did believe in the existence of demons but opposed torturing and executing supposed witches. In his writing he did believe there were approximately 7 million demons arranged in 1,111 legions of 6,666 demons each, although the Lutheran Church later felt that estimate of the demonic hoard was too low (Guiley, 2009). Scull (2015) notes that an understanding like Weyer's, that much of witch hysteria is in reality mental illness, was a common understanding during this time, including such notable humanists as Erasmus (1466-1536), and one that continues to this day. However, Schull (2015) notes that while overlaps occur between accusations of witchcraft, possession, and mental illness, they in reality are separate categories. For example, witchcraft is primarily centered around women, as has been shown possession is often involving women but not exclusively so, and mental illness occurs among all people, although those without funds or social standing have fewer supports.

The experience of mass hysteria, either in the form of exorcisms, witch trials, or ecstatic dance, seems to have occurred primarily in areas that would later become Protestant, including England, Germany and Sweden (Russell, 1972). James I of England/James IV of Scotland (1566-1625) became convinced of the power of witches after his fiancée, Anne of Denmark, was unable to complete her ocean journey to Scotland (Mastin, 2009). A subsequent trial was held against a witch who claimed to have kept Anne from sailing and prevented James from being able to make the journey himself. This led to the establishment of witch laws in Scotland and later England, and the king penned a book on witchcraft which included possession cases (James, 1597/2016). This event and the subsequent book influenced "The Scottish Play" by Shakespeare, *The Tragedy of Macbeth* (1623/2005).

Amsterdam in 1566 saw 30 children who were foaming at the mouth, convulsing, and eventually falling to the ground. Neither Lutheran clergy nor folk healers were able to exorcise them. However, when female witches among the community were discovered, the children reportedly recovered (Hoyt, 1978). Ireland, Spain, Italy, and Portugal, all predominantly Catholic countries, were less affected by witchcraft and heresy trials but are now seeing a dramatic increase in demonic possession and exorcism (Amarth, 1999; Kiely & McKenna, 2007; Wilkinson, 2007). An explanation offered by Wilkinson (2007) is that because these countries have a strong Catholic culture, personal problems are more acceptable if caused by a curse or demons, given that mental health issues continue to carry a stigma.

Oesterreich (1930) has ruled out false performances in most accounts of possession and exorcism in the Middle Ages and the Renaissance, claiming that these mass hysteria cases truly reflected the experiences of those suffering. Other mental health phenomena also have a contagious aspect, including self-cutting among the youth (Richardson & Surmitis, 2014), hysterical neurosis/neurasthenia as seen in the early days of psychiatry with Freud and Jung (Ehrenreich, 2009), and Personality Disorder (Loftus & Kitchum, 1994).

Mass hysteria continues to the present day, although not always related to possession. Hoyt (1978) documents a case of contagious itching at an elementary school in Berry, Alabama in 1973. At first, one or two young girls began to scratch themselves vigorously, but quickly classmates and then schoolmates began to break out and itch violently. A full investigation was done to see if the students were responding to a chemical exposure or other physical cause, which was ruled out. Pendergrast (2010) notes that students in the Special Education classes did not have any symptoms, perhaps because they did not realize they were expected to. Younger students who did not see any of the itching students also did not break out. Those most susceptible to the itching were female students, especially those who had other struggles (Hoyt, 1978; Pendergrast, 2010) The school was closed for the rest of the school year.

Hatchman (2015) contrasts two very distinct groups of students with similar outbreaks of hysteria or, diagnostically, conversion disorder. One group was impoverished Mexican schoolgirls, as well as some of the teachers and nuns, in an isolated Catholic boarding school in Chalco. The other was public high school students (all girls) in New York. Both displayed very similar symptoms as hysteria swept through both schools. Of course, other types of mass hysteria can be found, such as in the US a fear of Muslims that became especially fierce after the September 11 attacks in 2001. As I write there is also hysteria related to reported creepy clown sightings, including instances of schools being placed on temporary lockdowns (Teague, 2016).

Aaronovitch (2010) has written about the influence of various conspiracy theories upon the contemporary culture. Quoted at the end of the book is research done by Showalter (1997), who compares SRA, Gulf War syndrome, chronic fatigue syndrome, and alien abduction. A common pattern throughout these various complaints is an external identification for internal complaints, which may be physical or psychological suffering. Aaronovitch (2010), in commenting upon the research, notices gender differences; women studied by Showalter (1997) tend to have physical complaints. Men studied by Aaronovitch (2010) instead focused on conspiracy forces, a phenomenon labeled "hysteria for men" (p. 351). Another scholar, Brotherton (2015), disputes the gender difference in beliefs in conspiracy and points to a single study but does claim that numerous studies further indicate no difference between men and women's belief in conspiracies. In spite of the fact that Brotherton (2015) cites Aaronovitch (2010) on other areas of his research, there is no mention of Aaronovitch's gender-based findings.

Visual Display

Pictorial representations of demons become common in the Gothic period (roughly the twelfth to sixteenth centuries), at the same time that the arts moved from a formalized vision of Christ to a more human and suffering Jesus (Russell, 1972). Common portrayals in the Gothic period show Jesus with a greater sense of realism, and those around him are dressed in contemporary clothing for the time. The devil is shown as a hideous human, a vision of sin as disordered desire. Russell (1972) argues that these images reach their height with the nightmarish visions of Hieronymus Bosch (1450-1516). For Taylor (2007), looking at these images allows an understanding of the psyche of persons at that time, "They were objects of real fear, of such compelling fear, that it wasn't possible to entertain seriously the idea that they might be unreal" (p. 11).

The devil had often, in Europe, been associated with blackness, including men of African origins (Russell, 1972). This seems to connect with the Jungian (1976) archetype of the brute, an animal in behavior and drive. Russell (1972) points to the connection of white racism with this archetype, "animal strength, hairiness, great sexual potency, including outsized sexual organs" (p. 114) are all part of the reoccurring image of the demonic at this time. While distasteful, this form of racism did not yet manifest itself in the plantation-based chattel slavery of the American South. Black men or black devils show up often in trials of those accused of witchcraft, such as the Frenchmen Pierre Aupetit (executed in 1598) who described the devil as a black sheep who was greeted by a kiss on the anus, and Isaac de Auriran (executed in 1609), who described the devil as a large black man (Gulley, 2009).

Demos (2008) notes that in many of the witch trials in Puritan New England, black was not understood as describing African persons, of whom there were few in the community, but rather meant the indigenous inhabitants. However, the most famous witch trial of that time, the Salem trial, did begin with actions or accusations against an African woman from Barbados named Tabitha.

The overlapping of race and perceptions of evil continue to plague our culture, largely due to the unresolved conflicts stemming from the enslavement of Africans for centuries and the later systemic oppression of African Americans. The contemporary poet Claudia Rankine (2015), in commenting on the police shooting of Michael Brown, noted the officer found Brown frightening because he looked "like a demon" (n.p.). Rankine (2015) continues, "And I don't disbelieve it. Blackness in the white imagination has nothing to do with black people" (n.p.). It seems that there is a strong need within American culture to exorcise the demons of slavery, the attempted genocide of the indigenous communities, and ongoing discrimination in order for true healing to occur.

Understanding the Witch Craze

According to Stephens (2002), accusations about witchcraft in medieval Europe were inspired by two different groups of people, the illiterate lower class and the (significantly smaller) literate elite. For the lower class, the concern was about attempted destructive magic, (*maleficium*), which makes sense when placed within the context of the struggle for life at the time. Examples of protection from maleficium include protection from the "evil eye" and calling out to the moon during an eclipse to both help it out of darkness and ward off the magic that led to the celestial event (Kugel, 2011). White magic was often done by local providers, who were known in England as "Cunning" men and women (Demos, 2008). Levack (2013) notes concerns about *maleficia* (singular) were seen from the 15th century, with no reports of witches connected to maleficium or demon lovers before that time (Young, 2018). Baglio (2009) documents the continued focus upon it in modern-day Italy.

Stephens (2002) feels that accusations of possession and/or witchcraft from the elite were due to an unacknowledged anxiety over the existence of the supernatural world, an anxiety which would later result in the creative explosion that is the Renaissance. Demos (2008) notes that with the rise of the Inquisition, previous anxiety about individual magic changed to include the influence of Satan. Far from confined to history, these social anxieties continue into the present. Nash (1967) documents how in mid-century indigenous villages in Chiapas, Mexico, the community would informally try witches, often after they had been killed by those who felt the accused had harmed them or their family in some way.

For Russell (1972), witchcraft was closely connected with heresy. The common charges against medieval witches: that they killed and ate children, cursed their neighbors (both in person and in property), and engaged in sexual orgies, all mirror the charges against heretics of the same time (Russell, 1972) as well as those charges against Jews from Roman times to the present (Potok, 1978). Moss (2013) notes that these claims were also leveled in Roman times against "foreign" religions that were seen as possible threats to the state, including the rites of Dionysus. They predate Christianity (Russell, 1972), and appear in contemporary times in the debate over repressed memories and supposed Satanic Ritual Abuse (SRA) (Loftus & Kitchum, 1994; Ofshe & Watters, 1994), which has been called the best example of a modern-day witch hunt (Demos, 2008). However, as Carroll (2002) has documented, while Rome viewed all foreign unassimilated communities with suspicion, it was the Jewish community which continued to be plagued with these outlandish accusations, even into the modern age.

By 1000 CE or so, accusations of homosexual behavior at gatherings of witches become common as well (Russell, 1972). Eco (2007, 2011) has repeatedly satirized these claims in his historic novels that poke fun of conspiracy theories about the Knights Templar worshipping the demon God Baphomet, Freemasons engaging in a worldwide conspiracy of control, and *fin de siècle* occult practices. The classic text for medieval witch hunters, *Malleus Maleficarum* (translation, *The Hammering of Witches*) written by a Dominican friar in 1486, includes stories of witches being recruited by secret groups, being forcibly raped, and engaging in child sacrifices in their rituals (Demos, 2008). Members of the late Gnostic movement known as either Cathars or Albigensians were believed to meet in special meetings, known from the twelfth century on as a synagogue, which was later (in the middle of the fifteenth century) shortened to *shabbot* (Russell, 1972). Thus heresy, social control, and anti-Semitism became united in one word. It is interesting to note that literally underground rituals shrouded in secrecy, sometimes including bloodletting and even faked murders, were also a part of the worship of Mithra in the Roman world, a cult that had widespread popularity before the enforcement of Christianity as the official religion (Hale, 2009). Demos (2008) claims that the descriptions of the shabbot (or sabbot) helped to create a mental schema which allowed for the witch craze to gain strength, given it was a large gathering believed to include heresy as well as sexual deviancy.

Accusations of witchcraft continue in places throughout the world. Most curses or maleficia practices are socially condemned, and Guiley (2009) notes the forbidding of curses in the Christian tradition. Middleton (1967) documents how curses are used as a social enforcement tool among the

Lugbara tribe in Uganda and the Congo. Within that community, a clan head can curse those within the family in order to prevent unwanted behaviors, although there is a sharp distinction drawn from curses merely thought versus curses spoken.

While contemporary witchcraft in Africa is well documented (Linde, 2001; Stoller, 1989; Stoller & Olkes, 1987), other parts of the world also have seen evidence of witch belief. In the Indian state of Assam, 17 people were killed in witch hunts in 2011 (*The Economist*, 2012b). One survivor, Ranjita Basumatry, claims that it was jealousy that inspired her accusers, who attacked her and drove her family from their village. The article also gives a larger context to the assaults; not only is India undergoing significant social changes, but the state of Assam is in the midst of an independence movement connected to the largest tribal group, the Bodo. Witches, known as *dain* in Assam, are always female and born into their status, whereas men can become *ojha*, a learned role that fights black magic.

Reis (2013) notes that in Uganda, children often enact possession by evil spirits, which bears a significant resemblance to witch-children in other parts of the continent. Explanations for the frequency of this include dynamics after intense conflict within the culture and specific conflicts within the family system. Reis (2013) does argue that the process has potential for healing, but is also fraught with challenges. Adinkrah (2011) sees no value in the phenomenon of witch-child beliefs, but views it as a form of scapegoating family illnesses, death, or business failure. The complicity of members of the faith community, in this case both traditional and Christian in Ghana, is specifically cited and criticized by Adinkrah (2011).

In a study of a village in Nepal that experienced an epidemic of possessions associated with witchcraft, Sapkota, et al. (2014) note the following rates of co-occurring illnesses when compared to villagers with no possession symptoms: anxiety 68% (versus 18% in the control), depression 41% (versus 19% in the control), and most tellingly, PTSD 27% (versus 0% in the control). It seems clear that there was a cultural approach to handling distressing emotions.

The Standardization of Demonology

Wilkinson (2007) writes about Fr. Girolamo Menghi (1529-1609) who collected the existing writings about demons into a coherent whole, published in 1576 as *Flagellum Daemonum* or *The Devil's Scourge* (Menghi & Paxia, 2002). The text was widely reproduced and at times compiled with other writings such as *Malleus Malficarum* (Hardtke, 2015b). This urge to collect and compile information was one of the outcomes of the Enlightenment (Greenblatt, 2011). With or without the influence of the texts, if appears that exorcisms at the time remained common and approaches to the Rite differed widely (Hoyt, 1978).

The Roman Catholic Church published *The Roman Ritual* in 1614 (trans. Weller, 1952), a definitive collection of rites for the church. Included are 3 signs of demonic possession: inhuman strength, knowledge of foreign language, and knowledge of hidden objects. The impetus for a clearly defined collection of rites was part of the Catholic response to the Protestant Reformation, culminating in the Council of Trent (1545-1563). Demos (2008) notes an increase in witch trials and possession narratives as part of the experience of the Reformation as religious identity became "supercharged" (p. 51). The movement included a desire to clearly define what the Catholic Church was in opposition to Protestant beliefs (Cook, 2009). Before Trent, there was no standard rite for the liturgy, let alone for exorcism, although there had been widely used books that included various rituals (Salzmann, 2015). An exorcism handbook, the *Manuale Exorcismorum*, was published in 1626 by the Bishop of Antwerp, which included the Roman Ritual as well as some additional texts (Hoyt, 1978). A later Lutheran text, *Universal Lexicon*, was published in 1733 and kept the 3 signs, making them common for both (early) Protestants and Catholics (Midelfort, 2005). Lutheran acceptance of exorcisms did not come easily. While Luther presided over an exorcism (Hardtke, 2015), he also critiqued supposed demonic evidence presented during exorcisms of Catholic teachings such as purgatory (Scull, 2015).

Levack (2013) notes that Calvinist areas had significantly less emphasis on possession, such as in Scotland. This goes against the representation in the popular TV show *Outlander*, which includes a historically inaccurate *Catholic* exorcist in the Highlands circa 1740, long after the area had undergone significant influence of the Presbyterian faith (Delgado, 2014). Greenblatt (1988) notes how the more Calvinist wing of the Reformation movement in England tried to ban public exorcism as both an example of Roman Catholic practice and as public theatre, a form of religious performance. The Protestant de-emphasis on exorcism was not universal; Scull (2015) notes how an event in 1602 became a rallying point for the Puritans. A young girl, Mary Glover, was supposedly attacked by a witch. Her family, who were devout Calvinists, organized what are reported to have been effective exorcisms for the young girl and pushed for her tormentor, an elderly woman named Elizabeth Jackson, to be executed. Jackson's life was spared due to the witch laws no longer being enforced, but the story of Mary Glover would be repeated for a long period of time.

Jackson was defended by medical persons who felt she was not a witch but rather hysterical, an argument which was supported by the moderate wing of the Reformers in England.

Hoyt (1978) documents a very interesting career, that of the English Puritan exorcist John Darrel (1562-1607). He worked as an exorcist as well as a minister, placing the blame for the possessed people with area witches. This process began when he was a rather young minister. In 1586, Darrel unsuccessfully attempted to exorcise a 17-year-old girl, and then had a woman arrested as a witch. She was quickly released and Darrel was rebuked by the justice of the peace. 10 years later Darrel attempted to exorcise a young boy after he experienced hallucinations and would go into convulsions. An area woman confessed to bewitching the boy, but only after being tortured. She subsequently died in jail due to complications from the torture. Darrel claimed the exorcism was successful, but there is wide belief that the demonic voices heard during the rite were likely produced by Darrel. Darrel was asked for his expertise in a case where a young boy, Thomas Darling, was reported to have become possessed after being cursed by a witch who was bothered by his flatulence. The woman spent a year in jail (Guiley, 2009). William Summers of Nottingham, who was exorcised by Darrel after being caught engaging in bestiality with his dog (Guiley, 2009), accused 13 women of witchcraft, although he then recanted that position, only to recant his original recant (Hoyt, 1978). The situation was investigated by the Bishop of London, who had Darrel defrocked and jailed as a fraud. The evidence against him included testimony that Darrel had prompted Summers in the trial that included Darling (Guiley, 2009).

It appears that the devils that Darrel had named in the exorcisms would be referenced in Shakespeare's *King Lear* (Gibson, 2006), when Edgar pretends to be mad. In the play this is contrasted by Lear, who is mad but not due to supernatural reasons. Scull (2015) interprets this tension as indicating that Shakespeare had read some of the widely shared pamphlets of the time that were equally critical of both the Catholic and Protestant focus on possession narratives. The Anglican Church, in Rule 72, soon after forbade the practice of exorcisms without the Bishop's knowledge and approval (Hoyt, 1978). Guiley (2009) claims that this Rule dramatically decreased the number of exorcisms performed in England from that time onward although there is contradictory evidence about this (see below). A later Protestant reformer, John Wesley (1703-1791), who helped form the Methodist denomination, strongly believed in demonic possession and encouraged communal prayer and personal fasting as a way of handling the devil's influence. Scull (2015) notes that Wesley inspired a mixture of both acceptance and widespread ridicule.

It would be nice to think of the Renaissance as ending witch trials, but they actually increased at this time, in part because the printing press increased the ability to disseminate ideas about witches (Russell, 1972). For Taylor (2007), the rise in witch trials at this time was two-fold. For Calvinists, there was an active attempt to view all forms of ritual as a type of magic which needed to be cleansed. For Catholics (and to a lesser degree, non-Calvinist Protestants who included a liturgical aspect to their worship), there was a desire for clarified beliefs, enforced norms, and centralized power. Taylor (2007) notes that this era also included widespread upheavals due to socio-economic changes. This resulted in an emotional energy that needed outlets, be it through trials, battles, or the new-found "Protestant" work ethic. Within Judaism, no formal rite was created for exorcism, but this time period saw a similar increase in possession and exorcisms within various Jewish communities, paralleling Christian and Muslim experiences (Dennis, 2015).

From reviewing the literature, it would appear that England was a very popular place for exorcisms in the 16th and 17th centuries, as were many places throughout the continent. Hoyt (1978) documents how an English Jesuit, William Weston (1550?-1615), was tried and imprisoned in 1586 after performing a number of secret exorcisms. Fr. Weston appears to have acted against the advice of older priests (Pollen, 1912). It should be noted that the Jesuit religious order, and Catholicism in general, was illegal in England at the time. Therefore, Weston's behavior could be seen as a form of civil disobedience. There was widespread discussion of his actions among the Catholic underground of the time (Hoyt, 1978). Weston had spent considerable time in Spain where he was eventually buried. Spain was an enemy of England at that time, which included the support of a spy network composed of Catholic clergy (Cook, 2009).

Hoyt (1978) cites the case of a child, William Perry of Bilston, Staffordshire, who in 1620 claimed to vomit pins and feathers as well as to having black urine. It was claimed that these symptoms appeared only when a Protestant was present. Civil authorities witnessed the boy placing ink in his chamber pot and otherwise faking his possession. Upon questioning, it became clear that the entire episode was created by Catholic Jesuit priests to discredit the Protestant movement. Perry continued with his antics even after Catholic clergy attempted to exorcise the boy. The ruse was revealed when he would convulse to the first words of the Gospel of John in Latin but not Greek, a language he did not know (Langston, 2015).

Richard Dugdale (born in 1660) was another supposed possessed Englishman who underwent a year of exorcisms from 1689 to 1690 by Calvinist ministers. The long process was written about in a number of pamphlets, both those which agreed with the Dissenters and felt Dugdale was possessed, and those which supported the established Anglican Church and felt he was engaging in play acting, perhaps for the financial gain of his family (Lea, 2015). Davies (2015) references the case of George Lukins (1744-1805), who was prayed over by 7 Methodist ministers, even though his possession was widely believed to be a way out of working. Cappucci (2015b) notes how an exorcism done by George Fox (1624-1691), the founder of the Religious Society of Friends (Quakers), helped to spread the religious message of the new denomination in England.

Criticism of the widespread use of exorcism did occur within Catholic countries at this time. In 1583, the French Catholic bishops issued a statement that stated:

> before the priest undertakes an exorcism, he ought diligently to inquire into the life of the possessed…he should consult with wise, prudent and well-informed persons…Melancholics, lunatics and persons bewitched often declare themselves to be possessed by the devil. However, those people are more in need of a doctor than an exorcist. (Hoyt, 1978, p. 27)

That rather pastoral and therapeutic advice (i.e. medical examination, consultation, and an examination of the social contexts of the person) continues to sound like a balanced approach to dealing with those who complain of the phenomenon into the present day. This blending of medicine and faith was also seen in the influential book *The Anatomy of Melancholy* (1621) by the Anglican priest Robert Burton. In the text, Burton argues that melancholy may have demonic influences or may open up a person to the influence of the devil, yet he recommended medical attention in addition to prayer. It should be remembered that contemporary medical practice of the time, including bloodletting and purges, could be similar to an exorcism (see Scull, 2015).

Protestant Reformers who were disturbed by the continued Catholic influences in England's Anglican Church famously traveled to the American colonies to set up utopian communities based upon their "pure" (hence Puritan) theologies (Vowel, 2009). Sagert (2015b) writes about the trial of Dorothy Talbye (also written Talbie), a woman who killed her three-year-old daughter named Difficulty in 1635, after years of suffering from domestic violence by her husband. She was tried and found guilty of murder, a trial complicated by the fact that she claimed she had acted under the direction of God. The court claimed that it must have been demonic possession, although modern readers would be hard pressed not to see a pattern of mental health and domestic trauma behind her actions. The court stuck to Puritanical theories of law that indicated, based upon strict readings of the Old Testament, murder must require execution. Godbeer (2015) notes 78 documented possessions in the New England colonies in the 17th century, not including the witch trials, such as the notorious Salem trial which was the influence on Miller's classic play *The Crucible* (1955) and which was a later influence on films such as *The Witch* (Benskiet, et al., 2015) and *The Village* (Mercer & Shyamalan, 2004). Demos (2008) notes that while not all witch trials included possession stories, it was often a part of the understanding of witchcraft at the time. Explaining why the witch craze became so popular at that time is hard to identify in one simple explanation. Demos (2008) cites the vast literature on this subject and finds the argument that this society was experiencing significant challenges from outside forces, including significant conflict with French and Native peoples, as well as increased economic differences within the community.

Hoyt (1978) has commented that possession narratives fell out of favor among Protestants in England in the 19th century while still being popular among the Catholic minority. For example, a story is shared of the Catholic priest Fr. Edward Peach in the Birmingham Archdiocese exorcising an unbaptized woman after unsuccessful attempts by Anglican clergy. Peach at the time was attached to a "Mission church" originally established by Franciscans to expand Catholic ministry in the Midlands region of England, an effort that was in part a response to Irish immigration to the area (Catholic Women's League, 2010).

Lior (2015a) documents a change in thinking among the Jewish tradition in the 16th century in regard to possession with the introduction of the concept of the *dybbuk,* a possessing spirit that had human origins. There are various understandings of the dybbuk's origins, being either a ghost seeking refuge or a truly evil ancestor that must pay for sins. Most of the possessed persons were women and the possessing spirits male, with the act of possession often associated with a form of rape. An example of a dybbuk is shown in the opening scene of the Coen Brothers' movie *A Serious Man* (Brevan, Coen & Coen, 2009). Dybbuk possession still occurs in some Jewish communities. Lior (2015a) documents a contemporary rabbi in Israel attempting an exorcism of a Brazilian person via Skype. This form of negative possession can be contrasted with ibbur, a positive possession by a deceased teacher that can be sought by praying at the teacher's tomb, a practice still found in some Orthodox Jewish communities in Israel (Lior, 2015b).

Midelfort's (2005) study of the practice of exorcism in the late eighteenth-century Holy Roman Empire by Fr. Johann Joseph Gassner (1727-1799) shows that it was an incredibly popular healing ministry in the midst of a collapsing empire. Gassner was a controversial figure in his own time, dividing both Catholics and Protestants into those who believed in the possibility of possession and those who either rejected the possibility or held a degree of skepticism, often out of fear of mass hysteria. These arguments were put forward in many publications of the time. *The Economist* (2011) notes that the German-speaking world had been undergoing a media revolution since the days of Martin Luther (1483-1546). Henri Ellenberger (1970) identifies that the very beginning of modern mental health approaches occurred in a clash between Fr. Gassner and Franz Anton Mesmer (1734-1815), who used hypnosis and popularized the theory of animal magnetism, and whose name provided the origin of the term mesmerize (see also Crabtree, 1988; Midelfort, 2005). Weeks (1996) cautions against reading too much into the opposing views of either man, as many people of the time accepted multiple explanations for phenomena such as possession. Shenk (2001) draws out the evolution in thought from Mesmer's notion of animal magnetism to hypnosis, which then became a significant influence on Freud and psychoanalysis, although Freud ended up forgoing hypnotism for free association.

Moving away from a belief in literal possession were writers like the influential seventeenth-century English scholar Joseph Mede (1586-1639), who was an early encourager of authorship studies of Biblical texts and who attributed demonic possession to mental health concerns. Mede appears to have influenced John Milton and Isaac Newton (Thomas, 1971). Among German language scholarship, Johann Salomo Semler (1725-1791) is considered a significant figure in encouraging rational approaches to religious thinking and personal expression (Midelfort, 2005). Members of the French Enlightenment were very critical of traditional religious viewpoints; Denis Diderot (1713-1784) wrote a novel (published posthumously due to its scandalous nature) that addresses the topic. *La Religieuse* or *The Nun* (1796/1974) tells the story of a young woman compelled to enter a convent. The young nun later undergoes an exorcism that is compared to the pain of Jesus at death (as cited in Phillips, 2015b), as well as somewhat salacious unwanted advances from the mother superior.

The Enlightenment brought about a tension between those who held to a mechanical view of the world (which allowed little to no room for spirits) and those, often from the lower classes, who held onto traditional beliefs (Midelfort, 2005). This tension would spill over in later centuries as the clash of fundamentalism and modernity (Armstrong, 2001). It was not just Christianity that experienced this tension; the Jewish folk tradition of Hasidism was founded by Yisroel ben Eliezer (b. circa 1700-1760), who was an exorcist (Potok, 1978). This charismatic leader, better known as

Ba'al Shem Tov or the Besht, was working at a time when the educated elite in Judaism was moving away from belief in exorcisms and demons (Verter, 2000). There are a number of exorcism stories connected with the Besht, as well as stories that place an emphasis on healing rituals, including the use of amulets (Cappucci, 2015a).

Kemp and Williams (1987) document how belief in demonic possession steadily decreased in the Western world starting in the Renaissance. Porter (2002) noted historically how all forms of mental illness were first seen as spirit-based, then as building upon the work of Galen (b.130-210 CE) and the Hippocratic tradition as a result of bodily humors, and finally as either physical or psychological-biological-social in origin. Etiology is hardly without contemporary controversy (see, for example, Frattaroli, 2001). Oesterreich (1930) argues that spirit possession occurs in a society for two main reasons: the society believes in spirits, and people desire to communicate with them. Using this criterion, he argues that when a belief in spirits disappears, so do spirit possessions. Lewis (1986/2003) has noted that the counterculture of America and other Western cultures includes changing beliefs in the existence of an enchanted world and encourages trance states through drug use, although often without reference to spirits. Goodman (1988b) argues that those trance states are one of the reasons for an increase in belief in the possibility of spirit possession, although he cites no evidence for the claim.

In southwestern Germany near the Swiss border, two Lutheran pastors, Johann Christoph Blumhardt (1805-1880) and his son, Christoph Friedrich Blumhardt (1842-1919) became well-known for their work as exorcists (Winn, 2015a; Winn, 2015b). Initially the elder Blumhardt exorcised a man in his parish, not through the more traditional rites available, but rather with spontaneous prayer and fasting (Winn, 2015b). This led him to the conclusion that the power of God was breaking through in the present age and that many types of healing could be found through the laying on of hands. He then left his parish and founded a healing spa, ministering both to those with wealth as well as those who were indigent (Winn, 2015b). After his death, his son assumed the ministry but expanded from purely physical and spiritual healing to include a focus on social problems, such as the plight of workers during the Industrial Revolution (Winn, 2015a). Demonic enslavement meant, for the younger Blumhardt, not only possession but also militarism, racism, imperialism, and a focus on wealth. This brought him to join a Marxist party and to denounce Germany's part in World War I, which then resulted in his defrocking from the state church (Winn, 2015a). He is credited with influencing the "Confessing Church" of those Christian Germans who resisted the Nazis in World War II, such as Dietrich Bonhoffer (Winn, 2015a).

The Faust Story

While the story of Faust is not directly connected to possession, it bears some resemblance to the possession narrative. The story is perhaps best known to modern readers either from Christopher Marlowe's play, *The Tragical History of Doctor Faustus* (1604/1994) or two separate versions by the German literary genius Goethe (1808, 1832, trans. 1962) in which the character is known as Faust. In both writers' telling, Faust/us faces boredom and attempts suicide before making a pact with the devil for his soul in exchange for worldly knowledge, wisdom and experiences. In Marlowe's (1604/1994) version, the play ends with Faustus going to hell, although it is left to the reader/viewer of the play to imagine, as it occurs offstage. In Goethe's version (1808, 1832, trans. 1962), Faust is saved by the Virgin Mother and brought to heaven. It may be that the later influence of Romantic optimism was an influence on Goethe, as all of the earlier versions of this story involve Faust's damnation. One of the origins of this story is that of St. Theophilus, who sold his soul to the devil (or in other versions, to a Jewish witch) in order to secure a bishopric. St. Theophilus eventually received his eventual salvation with the intersession of the Virgin (see Radl, 2012).

There is evidence that this story has truly ancient roots. One current theory claims that this theme, labeled "The Smith and the Devil", dates back 6,000 years, predating written records (Flood, 2016). The story has had great staying power and was used as a critique of Soviet bureaucracy in Mikhail Bulgakov's (1966, trans. 2008) novel *The Master and Margarita*, and may have influenced the Rolling Stones in their song "Sympathy for the Devil". The Faust story also appears in Charlie Daniel's classic county song "The Devil Went Down to Georgia", released in 1979, as well as in both Washington Irving's story "The Devil and Tom Walker" (1824/1998) and "The Devil and Daniel Webster" by Benet (1937). Among the Quiché in Guatemala, there are stories of *win*, or shape shifters, who become such a creature through a similar dual with the devil. Saler (1967) described the process as:

> [One] who desires to become a *win* is said to sleep for nine nights in the cemetery, where he prays to the Devil. On the ninth night the latter appears and engages the man in combat with machetes or swords. If the Devil succeeds in inflicting the first wound, the man will die within seven days. If, on the other hand, the man first wounds the Devil, the latter will confer

> on him the power to become a *win*. Thereafter he returns frequently to the cemetery to transform himself into his nonhuman form, to commune with the Devil, and to feast on the bones of the dead. (p. 80)

The continued reproduction of this theme, over many centuries and in more places than it is worthy to mention, suggests that there is an aspect of dealing with the dark side of the self that continues to resonate.

There appears to be a real-life version of this story in the case of Johann Christoph Haizmann (1651/1652-1700), an Austrian artist who had reportedly sold his soul to the devil in two different contracts, one written in blood and one written in ink. This required him to have two different exorcisms, after which he joined a religious order and painted a church triptych of his experiences. A text of his story, as well as numerous ballads based upon it (Hoyt, 1978), was written a generation after his death. The whole story was commented upon by Sigmund Freud (1923), who felt Haizmann was likely schizophrenic. Freud rather characteristically classified the issue as having to do with Haizmann's unresolved issues with sexuality and his family, claiming that Haizmann's "road took him from his father, by way of the devil as Substitute Father, back to the devout Fathers" of the monastic enclosure and the Roman Catholic Church (Hoyt, 1978, p. 41). A modern mockumentary about the situation, with the film crew discovering ever-present satanic influences in their filming, is entitled *Searching for Haizmann* (Gordon & Meyer, 2003).

This storyline is also repeated in the story of Robert Johnson (1911-1938), the legendary bluesman who supposedly sold his soul to the devil at a crossroads in exchange for guitar playing skills. While the story is often repeated (e.g. Evans, 1971; Graves, 2008; Guralnick, 1998; Wald, 2004), in the radio program *RadioLab* (2007) there is a discussion not only of the historical roots of the story, but also its staying power as it continues to reverberate within the culture, long after Mr. Johnson's early and obscure death at the age of 27. Recent manifestations of the tale include an appearance of Johnson (referred to as Tommy Johnson, another blues musician who also is attributed to be the origin of the story) in the movie *O' Brother Where Art Thou?* (Coen & Coen, 2000) and in the novel *Reservation Blues* (Alexie, 1995), which compares the experience of African Americans and Native Americans as Johnson appears on the Spokane Indian Reservation, inspiring some young tribal members to form a band. Yonchak (2015) notes that the story has antecedents with Niccoló Paganini (1782-1840), an accomplished violinist whose virtuosity was attributed to demonic influence. Other historic figures are reputed to have had dealings with the devil, including the scholastic friar Roger Bacon (1219/1220-1292), who supposedly had a bronze head that could speak with the aid of a devil (Wall, 1905). It is interesting that the story developed as the historic Bacon, while a man of his medieval time, appears to have discouraged looking to supernatural sources for some natural phenomena in favor of natural understandings (Pye, 2014).

CHAPTER THREE

MODERNITY AND EXORCISM

Defining Modernity

When did modernity start? For C.S. Lewis, the writer of the Narnia series as well as a scholar of Medieval and Renaissance Literature, it was not until about 1830 or so, with the birth of the Industrial Revolution (Jacobs, 2005). Other scholars place the arrival of modernity at an earlier date. Harvey (1989) attributes Enlightenment thought, especially of the 18th century, with the birth of the modern. White (2006) places the birth of modernity at around 1600. For the Pulitzer Prize winner Greenblatt (2011), the process was connected with the humanists who rediscovered and popularized the thoughts of the pre-Christian classical world, thus beginning the Renaissance. For Manchester (1993), the process began with the "discovery" of the New World, which shattered older models of thought (see also Armstrong, 2014). Whatever the start, one way of understanding modernity is the shift to a material worldview as a majority view, away from an enchanted world influenced by spirits and spiritual forces. This definition is especially accurate for later modernity.

For Taylor (2007), modernity includes the tendency, as portrayed in Fyodor Dostoyevsky's novel alternatively translated as *The Possessed* or *The Devils* (1872, trans. 2009), to dismiss the miracle of life with the practical considerations of the group. This is exemplified in the novel when a midwife dismisses the newly-born as nothing more than an "organism" who may not be worthy of life. Dostoyevsky's story continues as nihilistic radicals are willing to kill others (and themselves) in a mistaken effort for social change. Thus, demonic influence is shown especially among those who are rejecting the spiritual for the material. For Halliburton (2010), modernity includes a discounting of smaller, regional, and cultural understandings and a subsequent replacement with universal explanations for the world, be it Science or the State. The example given is how in the Indian state of Kerala, psychic distress had been understood to be caused by specific regional spirits who are the source of possession; only to be replaced by either "anonymous" spirits or a more psychiatric explanation of symptoms such as "depression" or "tension". Harvey (1989) views modernity as an urbanizing process that increases the sense of alienation and individual isolation as a consequence of mass migration to large cities, which is a dynamic often seen in a globalized world and has been shown to lead to an increase in mass hysteria and belief in possession narratives (see chapter 2).

Modernity and Possession

Many modern thinkers automatically dismiss all reports of possession, especially in ancient literature, as an inadequate diagnosis that can better be explained now by psychological insights (Shermer, 2003). For example, Norris (2008) quotes the novelist Joyce Carol Oates in saying that, ". . . demonic possession—a primitive stage in our comprehension of mental illness we like to believe we've advanced beyond" (p. 37). Gabriel Garcia Marquez (1995) uses the belief by a young woman that she is possessed (when in fact she has rabies) as the opening of a forbidden romance that she has with her exorcist priest in the novel *Of Love and Other Demons*. Solomon (2001) quotes a friend, Eve Kahn, on the effects of schizophrenia on her father: "You understand where theories of demon possession come in, because someone had taken over my father's body. I was five years old and I could see it. I remember it very well. He looked the same but there was nobody home" (p. 82).

Spiro (1998) calls the scientific fallacy the belief that every phenomenon can be explained away in the mechanical-medical model. "There are dangers in reducing the experience of demonic possession to some supposedly more fundamental psychopathological condition, to neurosis, hysteria, psychosomatic disorder, and so forth" (Midelfort, 2005, p. 83). Increasingly, scholars are questioning the tendency to dismiss everything that is outside of our mechanical worldview. For example, Cohen (2002) has written that the placebo has become a medical slop sink, having everything poured into it in an attempt to dismiss the possibility of other types of agency and meaning-making. Csordas (2002) has acknowledged that to explain all types of physical illness in medical terms, especially if the suffering person would use other explanations, is to place our own worldview in place of their own. Ruth Harris, in her study of the supposedly miraculous healings in Lourdes, France (1999), sees these healings as examples of self-transformation, including a new approach to life. While many of the healings of Gassner and Lourdes can be explained, there are others which cannot. Even the ability to dismiss what is labelled "miraculous healing" has been brought into question by a medical doctor, Larry Dossey (2003).

America and Ecstatic Experiences

Kiev (1973) notes glossolalia and dissociative states occurred often amidst Methodist revivals during the First Great Awakening in the early 1700s in what was to become the United States, and may have helped to inspire the later revolution against the British. About one hundred years later there was a similar outpouring of religious fervor known as the Second Great Awakening, which was commented upon by the French visitor to the US, Alexis de Tocqueville (2000) in the 1830s (see Leon, 2000). While many at the time did not believe themselves to be possessed, some did, including the famed Confederate soldier “Stonewall” Jackson (Floyd, 1999). This style of religious energy is still experienced within the Pentecostal tradition, which appears to be experiencing a third wave of energy in the formation of new denominations such as Vineyard (Luhrmann, Nusbaum & Thisted, 2010). Woodward (2016) argues that a Third Great Awakening is happening now, including the rise of new denominations coupled with a significant disaffection with current religious structures, and a broad and inclusive spiritual focus. People who are experiencing spirit possession (as opposed to demonic possession) consistently report feelings of ecstasy as well as an experience of being outside of oneself (Lewis, 1989). This experience, Lewis notes, gives a degree of status to the participant, making it appealing to oppressed minorities, but possibly perpetuating unjust systems by providing a release mechanism for tension that might otherwise be directed at efforts to address societal injustice (Leon, 2000; Lewis, 1986/2003).

Spiritualism

Spiritualism as an international phenomenon appears to have a beginning around the middle of the 19th century. It tended to be characterized by an interest in communicating with the deceased, especially members of one’s family. Most writers date the beginning of this to the 3 Fox sisters in central New York, who claimed that rapping sounds heard in their home were made by ghosts. Their report achieved quick fame (Houdini, 1924/2011). The sisters lived in what is referred to as the “Burned-Over” district of New York, due to the Second Great Awakening beginning there, including the birth of several denominations including the Church of Jesus Christ of Latter Day Saints (aka the Mormons), 7th Day Adventists, and Jehovah’s Witnesses. The area was also a center for the Women’s Rights movement as well as communitarian socialists such as the Oneida Community (Wellman, 2000). Crow (2015) notes how women played a very prominent role within the Spiritualist movement. Spiritualist experiences are mentioned a great deal in the early American psychologist William James's classic *Varieties of Religious Experiences* (1901/2011).

Spiritualism did not just have an impact within the United States. Summers (1958) tells of a possession in 1850's France that has uncanny parallels with the Fox sister story, including rapping on walls, a point made in the text. Hoyt (1978) cites the story from Summers but does not include the reference to the Fox sisters. There were times that Spiritualism overlapped with more traditional versions of "ghost stories". An example would be "The Bell Witch", which was an early 19th century witch or ghost that haunted (depending upon the version of the story) either a slave plantation or a simple farm in either North Carolina or Tennessee (Ruickbie, 2015a).

Conservative Christian writers were very critical of the Spiritualist movement (Hayword, 2015). However, some denominations embraced the movement, such as the Shakers. Reece (2016) writes about how the adaptation of the spiritualist practices into Shaker communities brought new life into the celibate movement that had begun to see a decrease in membership. However, modern readers of the medium-delivered messages experience extreme discomfort at the stereotypical responses, especially when earnest Shakers were channeling disembodied indigenous spirits, as can be seen in the following passage:

> "Ho ho ho poor me poor me just from eternity
> Seeking seeking here for a crumb.
> Me fall upon my knee me trimmer at the sight,
> To see the shiney whites all marching in the light.
> Me poor Indian stand here in demidst
> leaning on my staff loaded down with sin & condemnation
> me beg entrance in some shiney white man
> me poor and needy
> me want to help my sin and make peace." (Reece, 2016, p. 44)

Critics of Spiritualism, such as Harry Houdini (1924/2011), the popular magician and escape artist, helped to bring about a decrease in the popularity of the Spiritualism movement by the time of the Depression (Crow, 2015). There does continue to be a small lasting presence; one of our receptionists in a clinic I work at is also a medium, and belief in contact with spirits is a common enough description among many of my clients as well as on television, with ghost-hunting shows being especially popular. Gallop (2005) states that about 1/3 of surveyed Americans have a belief in ghosts. The famed scholar of stages of grief, Elizabeth Kübler-Ross (1926-2004), became involved with the Church of the Facet of the Divinity. The religious practices included *séances* where physical entities of supposed otherwise disembodied spirits appeared and, on at least some occasions, had sex with attendees (Woodward, 2016). Spiritualist practice has continued in places such as Brazil among a variety of different religious groups (Dawson, 2015). Engler (2015) has shown how at least 2% of the Brazilian population self-identify with Spiritualist beliefs, and around 10% of Brazilians engage in some form of spiritualist-informed activities, such as attending study groups or *séances*.

Spiritualism was a major influence on what is often referred to as the New Age Movement, although there are other influences such as indigenous traditions from the First Nations of the Americas as well as utopian efforts which were also very common in the mid-1800s (Singler, 2015). Generally speaking, New Age thought does not believe in involuntary demonic possession and frequently places less emphasis upon evil forces than do many forms of Christianity, but the ability to channel other spirits is a common belief within the New Age Movement. One exception to the lack of emphasis on involuntary spiritual possession comes from Dr. Carl Wickland (1861-1945), a Swedish-born American psychiatrist who believed that many mental health complaints arose due to interference by disembodied spirits (Dollar, 2015). He developed a machine that produced a mild electric shock in order to jolt the spirit from the patient's body and into the waiting body of his wife Anna, who was a medium. It is interesting that even among contemporary spiritualists, this approach does not continue.

Fundamentalism and Pentecostalism

Cox (1995), in writing about current ecstatic experiences among Pentecostals and Charismatics, places the phenomenon less in a socio-economic context and emphasizes the existential dilemma in a Post-Enlightenment, disenchanted world. It is interesting that Cox places ecstatic experiences in a tension with fundamentalism, because these experiences are potentially authoritative, whereas within fundamentalism power is contained within formal structures and rigid understandings of key canonical texts (Armstrong, 2014). This tension is obvious when looking at fundamentalist Islam's tension with Sufism, the mystical and ecstatic tradition of Islam that includes the poetic description of becoming intoxicated by Allah (Armstrong, 2014; Lewis, 1986/2003).

While Pentecostal and fundamentalist Christians seem to have become bedfellows in the past several decades, they may not be too comfortable in that role. Fundamentalism is in tension with the modern world (Marty, 2000). Marty does not include some expressions of Catholicism in fundamentalism, in contrast to Cuneo (1999), who sees within neo-traditional Catholicism significant similarities with Protestant fundamentalism, although both sides would disavow such a comparison. While fundamentalism, evangelical Christianity, conservative streams within Roman Catholicism, and Pentecostalism share much in terms of theology and a basic worldview, fundamentalism stands out in opposition to much of the intellectual heritage of the Enlightenment (Marty, 2000). As Armstrong (2008) has pointed out, by insisting upon one type of interpretation of Scripture, namely a literal reading of the text, fundamentalism is also a symptom of modernity.

Contemporary Pentecostal expression would include not only some of the established denominations such as Assembly of God but also newer forms, such as Vineyard, which often meets in non-traditional settings such as gyms or malls, and owes at least some of its origins to the 60's era Christian Hippies known as the Jesus People (Luhrmann, Nusbaum & Thisted, 2010). Levack (2013) has noted that Pentecostals differ from previous enthusiastic sects like Methodists and Pietists in that there tends to be a lack of denominational oversight, although with the increasing acceptance of Pentecostals into new or existing denominations, that may change.

Catholicism and Modernity

The coming of the twentieth century was a time of serious wrestling within the Catholic Church in regards to modernity. The Pope at the turn of the century, Leo XIII (1810-1903), both accepted some aspects of the modern world (for example, labor unions) as well as rejecting others, like elections. His thoughts on modern life were mostly expressed in the influential encyclical (a letter to the bishops) *Rerum Novorum* (1891). There was still a tendency to clearly divide the world into an "us and them" mentality, such as in the encyclical *Humanum Genus* (1884). The text, which identifies the church with God's kingdom, lumps all the opposition to the church with a kingdom of Satan, which he associated with Freemasons and included democratic movements as well as the rising tide of Marxism. As a response to the position of the church, the professional prankster Marie Joseph Gabriel Antoine Jogand-Pagès (1854-1907), using the pen name of Leo Taxil, wrote a four-volume history of the Masons that associated them with Satanic rituals (Hause, 1989), a hoax that continues to have reverberations throughout the culture to this day. For example, Taxil's book has provided the basis for much of Eco's (2012) novel *The Prague Cemetery* and ended up being referenced in an interview I had with Fr. Tom, a contemporary exorcist (see chapter 9).

The same Pontiff, Leo XIII, in 1886 ordered the use of an exorcism prayer in all low masses after the formal conclusion of the service. These so-called "Leonine prayers", include a "Prayer to St. Michael". It is believed that the original writing was in response to the newly emerging Italian state's attempt to take possession of Papal land, but the prayer was later attributed to a vision in which Leo heard God give the devil power to destroy the church for a period of 100 years (see, for example, Fr. Saunders, 2003, for one example of this story). Often repeated in conservative Catholic circles with many variations, there is no version of this story discovered which pre-dates 1933, close to fifty years after the prayer was first published. This casts a degree of doubt therefore on the story (Bers, 1934). It is interesting to note with the creation of the Vatican State, the Leonine prayers were ordered to be said for the conversion of Russia, then under communist control. Salzmann (2015) notes that this prayer differs from most other exorcisms in that it is for a geographic area that is possessed or threatened, initially the Papal States, then Russia.

Modernity and Theology among Christianity

While attempts to modernize Christian theology go back to the early days of the Enlightenment (Midelfort, 2005), it became increasingly common in the 1960s among liberal theologians like Rudolph Bultmann (1969). For contemporary Christians, a difference can be drawn regarding demons and other spiritual entities. I would attempt to place such a divide on a continuum from liberals, who view ancient reports of demonic possession as outdated holdouts from a superstitious world or alternatively see it as a metaphor; to traditionalists (a category that includes fundamentalists, but is also broader), who tend to actively believe in the real presence of evil in this world and therefore acknowledge the possibility of possession, although they may differ on the prevalence of possession states. Liberals tend to interpret phenomena like demons as either "old myths" (Spong, 1994) or "more than metaphor" (Borg, 1995, 2001). David Smith (1982) has argued that metaphor and symbol, although related, are not the same. A symbol is a clear item which stands for something else (e.g. the cross for Christians). A metaphor is an "open-access route" (p. 67), which has an unpredictable quality.

Liberals appear to be struggling to find a way of integrating into a spiritual context the Enlightenment perspective that the world is mechanical, as in the case of Spong (1994), or a more post-modern shifting to include a both/and understanding (Borg, 1995, 2001). While exorcisms by liberal members of religious communities seem to be rare (Cuneo, 2001), McKanon does document how some counter-culture far-left radicals will perform the rite as part of public protest, including at places like the Pentagon (2011). Laycock (2015f) notes the use of exorcism in several poems by Allen Ginsberg (1926-1997) and by later poets and activists, including the neo-Pagan Starhawk (b. 1951) at US military bases and the World Trade Organization (WTO). These actions appear to be more symbolic than actual, which would correspond to the belief of liberals, who have accepted the Enlightenment tradition and tend toward a more mechanical understanding of the universe. Those who are engaging in these rituals also do not fit into traditional doctrinal categories. McKanon (2011) includes some, like the excommunicated Catholic priest Philip Berrigan and his brother, Dan, who remained a Jesuit until his death. Ginsberg (Laycock, 2015f) originally was a devout Jew and later embraced a hybrid of Tibetan Buddhism and Hindu practices.

Traditionalists view the world as still charged with spiritual forces. The split between liberals and traditionalists generally corresponds to the culture wars (Hunter, 1992; Williams, 2000; Wuthnow, 1988). The culture war argument is that the major divide within US culture is no longer geographic, racial, or socio-economic; rather it is centered on a belief system that transcends older categories like religious denominations. Traditionalists, such as conservative Christians, Jews, and Muslims as well as others, might join forces on cultural issues like abortion while liberals might form a broad coalition to work on environmental issues or poverty. Such clear divides are inherently tricky, as the upper example shows; there are increasing numbers of traditionalists who are engaged in environmental work, and there are hard questions for liberals to answer when faced with the depth of depravity of which humans are capable.

Modernity and Psychology

The revolution in psychological thought, which is an integral part of modernity, is due to the polarizing brilliance of Dr. Sigmund Freud (Ivey, D'Andrea & Ivey, 2012). Freud famously dismissed religious practices as forms of neurosis, a stance which Victor Frankl (1969, 1988) attributes to the overly materialistic worldview out of which he was operating. Kathleen Norris (2008) notes the effects of this belief on Freud and disciples, "Belief in the efficacy of therapeutic methods is such a part of American culture that for many, psychology has replaced traditional religion. Some are tempted to regard religion itself as just another form of therapy, and an inadequate one at that" (p. 94). In researching the origins of psychology, Westerink (2014) notes the religious roots of Freudian psychoanalysis as well as earlier understandings of mental health issues such as neurosis and hysteria. The original Freudian diagnosis of hysteria has since been broken down into Histrionic Personality Disorder, DID, and Somatization Disorder (Mays, 2008).

Pattison (1973) has argued that while the first half of the twentieth century was characterized by hostility between psychology and religious perspectives, the second half of the century included at least a dialogue between the two ways of viewing the world. The text offers a case study from his experiences of working with the Yakima tribe in Washington State. Mary, a high school age female adolescent, came with her mother complaining of hearing voices, seeing ghosts, and feeling as though the ghosts were trying to choke her. She would often appear in a daze, and reported that she often saw blood that she blamed on murders the ghosts had committed. In doing the mental health assessment, Mary's mother stated that Mary's grandfather was a tribal shaman who had stated that his gifts would be passed on to a grandchild. However, since the grandfather's death, the family had converted to Christianity and did not practice the traditional ways anymore. According to Mary's mother, the "shaman to be" had to struggle against the spirits in order to gain healing power. Mary refused to participate. Pattison helped the family arrange a traditional healing ceremony similar to an exorcism to send the ghosts away. What was interesting is that the family knew of the appropriate ceremony; they needed permission from a Western healer in order to proceed. Personally, I worked briefly with a Native American woman who felt called to be a medicine woman but refused, and reported being haunted by spiritual presences in a manner similar to Mary's.

Christian Exorcisms in the 20th Century

In general, the primarily immigrant Catholic communities in the US during the 19th and early 20th centuries downplayed exorcisms, in part due to the attempt to fit into the mainstream of American culture (Koningisor, 2011). One noted exorcism done by a Catholic priest in the US in the early 1900s (Kiely & McKenna, 2007) was of a woman known simply in their text as Mary X, who underwent an exorcism in 1928. She had been abused by her father and her mother had killed several of Mary's siblings, yet the authors oddly suspect it was only after the deaths of both parents that demons appeared. One of the demons was her father's mistress, named

Mina. It seems likely that Kiely and McKenna (2007) are describing the exorcism of Anna Ecklund, a young woman whose experiences with exorcisms occurred both in 1908 (in Wisconsin) and 1928 (in Iowa) under a Capuchin priest named Theophilus Riesinger. It is reported that he had exorcised 22 people throughout his career (Hoyt, 1978).

In the version recounted in Crabtree (1997a), which is from a German text translated into English, the information is slightly different from that reported in Kiely and McKenna (2007). For example, Crabtree (1997a) reports that it was Mina who had probably aborted her unborn child and that her father had attempted an incestuous relationship with Anna. The text, which Crabtree quotes, has a number of paranormal events as part of the exorcism, including Anna levitating off the bed and hanging onto the wall. It is even more interesting that Hoyt (1978) claims Mina is an aunt of Anna (as well as the mistress of her father), and the initial possession was caused by Mina casting spells over the herbs in Anna's food.

Much later in time, the Austrian-born Jesuit Karl Patzelt achieved a degree of fame or notoriety from exorcisms he performed in the Los Angeles Catholic diocese immediately before and after the release of the film *The Exorcist* in the 1970s. His work ended up receiving national attention in both *Time* and *Newsweek* (Hoyt, 1978). Within the obituary it is reported that he was called in for more exorcisms until a change in the bishop of the diocese resulted in him no longer having that role (Pasternak, 1988). A fellow priest claimed that "he got fooled by a lot of people" (Pasternak, 1988). It is interesting that not only was Fr. Patzelt an immigrant but he also was a priest of the Byzantine Rite, a form of Catholicism that looks much more like Russian Orthodox worship than the Latin Rite (Cook, 2009).

In the early 20th century, Pentecostals frequently performed exorcisms or deliverance ministry, then the practice faded as the movement integrated into society, although it is still practiced in some Pentecostal churches (Cuneo, 2001). Many Pentecostals (and traditionalist Christians in general) also have a belief in spiritual warfare. Verter (2000), in defining spiritual warfare, notes that it is a belief that an individual or group is actively fighting Satan and other demons that are responsible for illness and social disruption. Well known Pentecostal figures like Oral Roberts engaged in deliverance ministries and encouraged the ideas of spiritual warfare. Frank Peretti (2003) encouraged the view that demons are engaged in a serious conflict over the soul of the world and appears to have a wide readership among conservative Christians, popularizing the view of a spiritual war. C. Peter Wagner is one writer who differentiates three types of spiritual warfare; challenging demons released by Occult practices, casting out individual demons, and challenging territorial powers that control an area (Wise, 2015).

In the 1970s, there was a new movement, known as Charismatic, Renewal, or neo-Pentecostal (Quebedeaux, 1983; Blumhofer, 2000), that spanned Protestant and Catholic churches (McGuire, 1982). In an attempt to return to a style of religion that was closer to the early Christian church, Charismatic worship is characterized by emotive worship and a renewed emphasis on spiritual matters (Neitz, 1987). A common but not exclusive example of that emphasis includes speaking in tongues, which is officially known as glossolalia (Werse, 2015b).

Some Charismatics included exorcism/deliverance as part of their spiritual practice (Cuneo, 2001). One such person in the United Kingdom was Reverend Christopher Neil-Smith, who popularized the practice and achieved a degree of fame for his ministry, especially after the popularity of *The Exorcist* (Hoyt, 1978). For Catholics, this could be a touchy issue, as a full exorcism can only be done by a priest and must be authorized by the local bishop, a rule going back to the Council of Laodicea in 363 CE (Kiely & McKenna, 2007). A solution was created that differentiated full possession, which would require an exorcism, from demonic oppression, which could be addressed by any baptized Christian using deliverance, a word often used in non-liturgical Protestant forms of exorcism (Cuneo, 2001). For example, Francis MacNutt (2009), a former Dominican order Roman Catholic priest (until he married the psychologist Dr. Judith McNutt without dispensation from the church), frequently engaged in deliverance work. My mother, who was active in the Charismatic renewal, remembers how closely healing was connected to belief in demonic oppression and deliverance ministry (see also Grady, n.d.). Contemporary Catholic Charismatics tend to view prayers for healing as occurring in four (non-exclusionary) areas: physical, psychological, spiritual, and deliverance/exorcism (International Catholic Charismatic Renewal Services, 2007).

Current Pentecostal ministries are expanding the exorcisms/deliverances performed (Cuneo, 2001; Kiely & McKenna, 2007), with some exorcising demons that could be understood by outsiders in metaphoric, moral, or medical terms. Derek Prince (1915-2003), for example, differed from the dominant view within Pentecostalism in the belief that Christians can be possessed (or at least oppressed) by demons after his own experience with depression (Bradnick, 2015). His 50 or so publications helped to spread the notion of deliverance ministries, as he took on the "demons" of caffeine, gossip, masturbation, and cosmetics. He also viewed Tourette's syndrome as demon-originated (Kiely & McKenna, 2007). Tourette's, characterized by involuntary movements and sounds, which may include obscene statements, has historically been seen as demonic but later, under psychoanalytic theory, as a consequence of masturbation, and of course is now understand as a medical disorder (Germiniani, et al., 2012). Frank and Ida Hammond (1973), a west Texas couple in a deliverance ministry, include demons of mental illness as well as vegetarianism (Kiely & McKenna, 2007), and are considered to be some of the most influential in promoting the idea of deliverance to the wider Charismatic movement. Apparently, the movement had achieved a degree of widespread cultural acceptance; Hoyt (1978) documents the public exorcism of a woman with multiple personalities at a pharmaceutical conference in Honolulu by the Baptist pastor Bill Smith, although I could find no other evidence for this very odd event.

The practice of evangelizing to gay and lesbian persons from a conservative Christian perspective began as a response to the newly energized LGBT movement after the Stonewall Uprising in 1969, an occasion widely seen as the start of the public push for greater acceptance (Laycock, 2015d). This is the same rough timeframe as the rise in deliverance ministries, which has resulted in a new hybrid of gay exorcisms, a practice that is mentioned in a seminal deliverance ministry text *Pigs in the Parlor* (Hammond & Hammond, 1973).

Popular Music

Yonchak (2015) documents how Western popular music has played upon older generations' anxieties since the stories of bluesmen who sold their souls to the devil like the aforementioned Robert Johnson (1911-1938). Some, like Eddie James "Son" House (1902-1988), left sacred music to pursue a career in the blues, while others left popular music to energize sacred song, such as Thomas Andrew Dorsey (1899-1993), who helped popularize Gospel music. However, it was the transition of African-American rhythm and blues into (mostly) Caucasian rock n' roll, beginning in the 1950s, that showed how fear of the "devil's music" was connected with underlying racial anxiety. One early example was "Screamin' Jay" Hawkins (1929-2000), who would perform his hit "I Have a Spell on You" as an African Witch Doctor. Hawkins was able to connect the older generation's racist connotations of a tribal African with sexual anxiety and make a living out of it.

Padrun (1995) has shown how religious images have been used by performers who tend to emphasize a sexual aspect to the symbols, such as Madonna (b.1958) and the recent sexually suggestive exorcism that Nicki

Minaj (b. 1982) performed at the Grammy Awards in 2012 (Channey, 2012). Darker demonic images have long been used in heavy metal since the English band Black Sabbath came out with their eponymous album in 1970, naming themselves after the Satanic Mass. Frequently, occult connections or references are attributed to metal artists. This includes Alice Cooper (b. 1948), who supposedly got his name from a Ouija board controlled by an executed witch (a story that he has denied, see BBC, 2009) and KISS, whose band name supposedly refers to being "Knights in Satanic Service", although that story has had no actual verification (Snopes, 2011). Other contemporary artists willfully play up the supposed demonic connections of the genre, including *Ghost*, a Swedish band that uses Gregorian chant with demonic names substituted and whose lead singer performs as a satanic anti-Pope (Yonchak, 2015).

The Power of Film

Cinematic representations of possessions as well as hauntings go back to early silent films. The first known film that addressed possession was a Danish film *Häxan*: *Witchcraft through the Ages* (Christensen & Christensen, 1922). Other early films include the Polish film with a Jewish theme, *The Dybbuk* (Waszynski & Mayflauer, 1937). It is worth noting that the prevalence of possession stories continues, and in fact has increased, while participation in religious communities has decreased. The use of religious images, even without the actual presence of a figure with religious authority, suggests the continued power of spirituality in an age when systems and structures such as denomination have ever less social and personal influence (MacLeod, 2015b).

The film *Constantine* (Adler, Aguilar & Lawrence, 2005) presents an interesting take on the possession narrative. In the film, the title character is able to identify possessed persons as well as the general presence of angels and demons. He attempts to engage in an exorcism of a possessed woman, Angela, who is frustrated that her sister, who died via suicide, cannot be buried in a Catholic cemetery. Constantine fails and commits suicide himself, which prompts Lucifer to retrieve his soul and somehow return the hero to Earth and to a healed Angela. The themes of frustration with existing power systems (be they Divine or ecclesiastical) seem to be part of the appeal of the film (and the comic book that the movie draws from)

The married couple, Ed and Lorraine Warren have made a career of lay demonology, being involved in ghost hunting and publicizing their findings in a variety of ways (Morehead, 2015b). They have written books such as *The Amityville Horror* (Anson, 1977), which was made into a movie (Arkoff

& Rosenberg, 1979) and then remade (Bay & Douglas, 2005). Guiley (2009) notes numerous lawsuits involved in the case, including those filed by the family that had previously owned the supposed haunted house and by a priest who insisted he did not bless the house, in spite of claims that he had done so. Other films inspired by the Warrens include *The Haunting in Connecticut* (Brooks & Cornwall, 2009) and *The Demon Murder Case* (Clark & Hale, 1983). The latter involved an unusual criminal trial where the defense used the argument that the murderer could not be convicted because he was possessed (Morehead, 2015a). It was not a successful defense. Cuneo (2001) notes how the couple connected many people to Catholic priests who were willing to perform exorcisms on the sly, without a bishop's knowledge. In one case, they were involved in bringing an English man, Bill Ramsey, to the States to be exorcised by a bishop, as Mr. Ramsey believed he was possessed by a werewolf demon (Morehead, 2015d). One of the exorcists interviewed in chapter 9, Laurene Gomez (2017), began her career due to the influence of the Warrens.

As mentioned in the introduction, the publication of the novel *The Exorcist* (Blatty, 1971), and the enduring fame and influence of the film version in 1973 (Blatty & Friedken; see also Blatty, 1974), brought images of demonic possession and exorcism to a much wider American audience than simply traditionalist Catholics and Pentecostals. Allen (1993), a journalist, researched the original case that inspired the book and movie. The child who was possessed is a boy called "Robbie". Allen places the situation within the context of racial tension over housing desegregation in the neighborhood in which Robbie lived in post-World War II suburban DC, and then St. Louis, where the exorcisms actually took place (a surprising fact given the prominence of the location of DC in the film). Specifically, the symptoms of possession began shortly after a beloved aunt died. Allen (1993) further raises the question of possible sexual abuse. Robbie would display revulsion at the station of the cross when Jesus is stripped. However, no evidence was ever put forward to indicate that he had been abused. MacLeod (2015a) notes how many of the lurid events that became key to the images of the novel and film, such as projectile vomiting and levitation, did not appear in the case of "Robbie". Ruickbie (2015b) notes the likely existence of a conversion disorder in "Robbie", but does not rule out possibilities such as poltergeist activities or other parapsychology.

The Exorcist book (1971) and subsequent film (1973) were written by a Lebanese Catholic immigrant, William Blatty. He also wrote a sequel to the book entitled *Legion* (1981), and helped write and direct the third sequel *The Exorcist III*: *Legion* (de Haven & Blatty, 1990). Blatty had no role in the first movie sequel, *The Exorcist II*: *The Heretic* (Boorman & Boorman,

1977), which has been called one of the worst films of all time (Leeder, 2015). Blatty identified one goal of his work was to promote Catholic thought in the culture at large, and in fact he recently sued his alma mater George town (which is also the setting for the film) for diverging from their Catholic mission by having pro-choice speakers on campus, in spite of the notion of academic freedom and the importance of students hearing a variety of viewpoints (Desmond, 2014).

Soon after the film, Malachi Martin (1921-1999) released a bestseller *Hostage to the Devil* (1976), which showed six sensational exorcisms and claimed a worldwide satanic conspiracy. Martin was a Jesuit who, in the aftermath of Vatican II, was released from his vows as a member of the order but not from his vows as a priest (Phillips, 2015). He was also a traditionalist Catholic, especially in his later years (Cuneo, 1999, 2001). Martin's writings tended to be conspiracy-minded, including the claim that his own former religious order, the Jesuits, were trying to take over the world (1987). In a very odd word of support, the psychiatrist M. Scott Peck (2005) called Martin "the biggest liar I have ever met" (p. 5), and dedicated the book that contains the quote to Martin. While Martin (1976) has some very solid recommendations in dealing with people who believe themselves to be possessed, such as the necessity of understanding possible physical and psychological origins, he also writes about wild events during the exorcisms (i.e. levitation, flying objects and the like) that are unreported in other contemporary exorcisms, except of course in the movies.

An Irish documentary was made about Martin called, like his famous book on exorcisms, *Hostage to the Devil* (Stalker & Marro, 2016). The film includes numerous interviews with those who knew Martin, mostly on a positive note. One exception was a fellow former Jesuit, William Kaiser, whose criticisms of Martin included the fact that Martin had an affair with Kaiser's wife. The saga of the affair constitutes the second half of Kaiser's memoir *Clerical Error* (2002), which is an intriguing book in that it also involves Kaiser's voluntary psychiatric commitment with paranoid schizophrenia, which has cast some doubt on his claims of Martin's infidelity. In general, the film ignores that fact that Martin's exorcism activities were with those who had broken from the Roman church after Vatican II, such as traditional Catholics like the Society of St. Pius X (also known as SSPX), and later included some who broke away from SSPX to form a more traditional denomination, in this case the Society of St. Pius V (SSPV). Both practice a pre-Vatican II Latin Mass and both have spilled much ink (or, in this digital age, many pixels) with criticisms of each other.

Glimpse of the Devil

Peck had already attracted attention when he, at that time a well-respected psychiatrist, wrote *People of the Lie* (1998). In the book, Peck argues that physical manifestations of evil do exist and that some people are possessed. He also admitted that he had performed two exorcisms, a revelation that was met with great acceptance among exorcists, many of whom viewed psychiatry as a modern opponent of their work (Cuneo, 2001). In *Glimpse of the Devil* (2005), Peck describes the exorcisms which he performed in the 1980s. His outlook and approach toward exorcisms come directly from Martin (1976), a fact which Peck readily admits. What is odd about the book is how little Peck (2005) further references the vast literature on the subject except to criticize Cuneo (2001) and mention some of his own (Peck's) previous works.

The first possessed client, a woman named Jersey, is a wife and mother who reports hearing voices that are getting louder and more intrusive. Peck (2005) dismisses schizophrenia or other forms of psychosis without going into his rationale, in spite of the fact that the voices continue even after the exorcism. He further dismisses Multiple Personality Disorder (MPD; now Dissociative Identity Disorder), in spite of the existence of distinct alters in the voices that Jersey hears. One of the voices, the final one to be manifested in the exorcism, is that of Lucifer. This leads Peck (2005) to the claim that all manifestations of possession are directly related to Satan, a stance which puts him at odds with Martin (1976) and most other exorcists, although as mentioned in chapter 2 this is consistent with a reading of the Gospel of John.

In the second exorcism, Peck (2005) is working with another woman, this one by the name of Becca. While Jersey was a stay-at-home mother, Becca is a high-rolling investment trader working with her husband, who is controlling and abusive. She too hears voices, as well as engages in self-cutting and long stretches of sun-bathing (which eventually leads to fatal melanoma). The cutting seems particularly interesting, in part because Becca, who is ethnically Jewish and was somewhat observant until she married her husband, is using WWII-era Nazi knives to do the cuts. Peck (2005) ignores the existing literature about self-cutting, if not when he was working with the client, when he was working on the manuscript (e.g. Walsh & Rosen, 1988; Miller, 1995; Levenkron, 1998) and places the blame for this behavior on Becca's possessed state. The exorcism is, in the end, rather unsuccessful, with Becca breaking off contact until word gets to Peck (2005) that she has died after failing to treat her cancer.

The book *Glimpse of the Devil* (2005) shows a high degree of similarity between the two clients who are possessed. Both experienced abuse from a young age, consistent with the population that experiences dissociative disorders as well as Borderline Personality Disorder (APA, 2013). Both became interested in expressing their own spirituality early, which fits with their developmental stages (Sigelman & Rider, 2009). Jersey, as an adolescent, expressed interest in the spiritual works of Edgar Casey (2004). Becca as a youth carried around a book of woodcuts, *God's Man* (Ward, 1978), which pictorially describes a Faust story in wordless woodcuts. For Peck (2005), these explorations of spirituality outside of accepted churches open up the two women to demonic possession. This is interesting because Peck himself had a long spiritual journey, one that ended in a rather loosely defined Christianity of a liberal sort, except for his conviction of the real presence of evil (2005). However, throughout the book, Peck seems to be obsessed with doctrinal clarity, accusing the demons possessing the women of heresy, a charge that is common not only in Martin (1976) but also throughout Western history (Russell, 1972). Using the criteria in the DSM-3 (APA, 1980), which would have been current when Peck was seeing his patients, it seems as if the both would meet the criteria of MPD, a fact which is not mentioned in the text.

Perhaps I am being unduly hard on Peck, and *Glimpse of the Devil* (2005) appears to have been written soon before his death. His early works are often well respected and are found on many a bookshelf, including those of mental health professionals, although *Glimpse* (2005) appears to be little read. However flawed the writing, it cannot be ignored that the two exorcisms occurred well before he wrote the book and he engages in behavior strongly recommended against, including incomplete differential diagnosis. It is unclear from the text how much either Becca or Jersey identified with the possession until the ritual really begins. In the end, neither appears to get much help from it.

The Increase in Contemporary Exorcisms

Cuneo (2001) claims exorcism/deliverance has been more widely practiced in the last 25 years than at any other time in US history. For Catholics, officially endorsed exorcisms were not common until the mid-1990s. Before then, the practice was mostly restricted to a small group of maverick far-right priests, often without the Church's suggested psychological testing for patients (Cuneo, 2000). Among Charismatics, popular writers on exorcism include Don Basham (1971), Hammond and Hammond (1973) and Francis MacNutt (2009), who advanced that Christians cannot be possessed but can have an indwelling demon or be demonically afflicted or oppressed, requiring deliverance (Laycock, 2015e). MacNutt claimed that between one-third to one-half of people are in need of deliverance, although the need for a full exorcism is rare (Bradnick, 2015).

Robert Pelton (1979) writes about an exorcism performed by a Holiness pastor and his wife, with a Baptist preacher and a Catholic priest in attendance, as well as observation provided by a psychologist, a psychiatrist, and three nurses. The grouping seems odd, as theologically it would be difficult to imagine such a theologically diverse team agreeing, let alone the cost at present of having such a team observe the situation. Perhaps it is telling that a current viewing of Pelton's website does not list the book (presumably it is out of print). He is a very prolific author with a current focus on the religious belief of the founding fathers, as well as cookbooks from the Revolutionary and Civil War. He did not respond to inquiries about the 1979 text.

Cuneo (2000, 2001) connects the rise in deliverance ministries in the 1970s and 80s to a shopping mall approach to spirituality: the ritual occurs, "In the brightly-lit, fulfillment-on-demand culture of the post-60's America. It could be engaged in as often as anyone wanted and for virtually any reason under the sun" (Cuneo, 2001, p. 244). Most exorcisms appear to be performed in private by pastors and Christian therapists, with some done *en masse* in auditoriums (Cuneo, 2000, 2001).

The rise in exorcisms seems to be tied to the fear of the occult. From 1983 through to 1993, there was a Satanism scare in the US (Richardson, Best & Bromley, 1991). More theologically conservative Protestants like Charles Kraft (1997, 2010) and C. Peter Wagner (2011) began deliverance ministries tied to fighting what was described as Satanic values. There was also a widespread belief in Satanic Ritual Abuse (SRA) that was popular at this time, fueled in part by the mental health community (see Demos, 2008). In an interview with Cuneo (2001), Dr. John Kelly discusses how he has treated many people who had memories of SRA. He does not believe that many of these memories are based in fact. However, he does state that "the memories might convey a potentially helpful therapeutic message to the person" (p. 211). Poole (2015) traces some of the origins of the "Satanic Panic" (p. 143) to England, which saw significant worries of desecration of graves and a heightened interest in the occult starting in the 1960s, when more and more people were leaving organized religious activities, including the established church. It should be noted that no external evidence of such widespread SRA was ever discovered (Bottoms, Shaver & Goodman, 1996). Ruickbie (2012) has documented how currently Botswana is experiencing a contemporary fear of Satanic influences, including high ranking government ministers examining the school system for signs of the devil.

Contemporary Harmful Exorcisms

Hoyt (1978) documents the beatings and eventual death of three-year-old David Weilbacher by a small cult in Yakima, Washington. After he died they hid his body in the back of the house for months (The Bulletin, 1976). The case of the British couple Michael Taylor (b. 1941) and his wife Christine (1941-1974) is cited by Ruickbie (2015c). Both were involved in a local Church of England charismatic prayer group, and Michael began to have very strong sexual feelings toward a female lay leader of their group, as well as a belief that another member was a Satanist. Soon Michael's behavior became steadily more erratic, but instead of referring him for mental health care for his deteriorating condition, he was given a very violent exorcism, including being restrained and having crosses forced into his mouth. The next day he killed his wife and mutilated her body. In an inquest held after the trial, the psychiatrist William Trethowan conjectured that the previous exorcism had created a "hysterical pseudo-psychosis" (p. 338). The publicity from the trial resulted in the Church of England revising exorcism policies requiring exorcists to be trained, authorized by the bishop, and done with consultation from medical professionals. Furthermore, it was required that those who had undergone an exorcism be scheduled for follow-up pastoral care (Ruickbie, 2015c).

Hoyt (1978) documents a 16-year-old Swiss girl, Bernadette Hasler, who was beaten for the sin of *Teufelsbuhlschaft*, that is sex with the devil. She died the next day. One of the people responsible for her death, after release from prison, was again convicted of killing a person in the midst of an exorcism. She has since been confined for life in a mental hospital (Hardtke, 2015). Both Goodman (1981, 1988b) and Kiely and McKenna (2007) write about Anneliese Michel, whose life is the basis for the film *The Exorcism of Emily Rose* (Derrickson, Boardman & Flynn, 2005) as well as *Requiem* (Putz & Schmid, 2006), and *Anneliese: The Exorcist Tapes* (Prest, 2011). In 1976, the young German woman was subjected to 10 months of weekly exorcisms after having epileptic fits. She also appears to have been anorexic and stopped eating altogether before her untimely death. The bishop and two priests who were involved were sentenced to 6 months in prison for negligent homicide, although the sentence was later commuted to 3 months. When reviewing the tapes from the exorcism sessions, Goodman (1981, 1988b) notes that after Michel had been prescribed Tegretol to help control her seizures, her glossolalia decreased, possibly preventing her from accessing the altered states of consciousness that were helping her to deal with her psychic pain. Modestino and Halloran (2015) note that the priest involved had a number of mental health concerns, including a history himself of schizophrenia and odd behavior during the police interview, suggesting a schizotypal personality disorder. In an attempt to address the death, the German Catholic bishops crafted an alternative text to the traditional rite of exorcism and encouraged the Vatican to consider their changes in the official universal revision of the Rite, an attempt that was unsuccessful (Hardtke, 2015). Guiley (2009) claims that more recently German Catholic bishops have questioned the need for an official revision of the exorcism rite given that they would not grant the authority to use the ritual within their dioceses.

A Romanian convent was the site of the death of a 23-year-old nun, Maricica Irina Cornici (1982-2005). Raised as an orphan, she was systematically abused throughout her life. She visited the convent where a fellow orphan whom she knew was living, and even before fully entering into the community she had a psychiatric break and was hospitalized and diagnosed with "early schizophrenia", what might be labeled now as schizophreniform disorder (APA, 2013). After her psychiatric medication had run out, she began to hear voices (Nicole & Manolache, 2015). No further medical treatment or psychiatric services were sought for her mental health concerns. Instead she was tied to a cross, had a rag stuffed in her mouth, was denied food and water, and died of asphyxiation and thirst. The convent was closed and the presiding Orthodox priest, Daniel Corogeanu, was sentenced to 7 years in prison (Cuneo, 2001). Nicole and Manolache (2015) note that the Romanian Orthodox Church bans exorcisms and attributes the incident to folk traditions and an institutional structure that had yet to adjust to the collapse of the Communist dictatorship. This incident became the basis for a Romanian film *Dupa Dealuri*, which was released to English language audiences as *Beyond the Hills* (Mungiu, 2012). A Russian Orthodox saint, John of Kronstadt (1829-1908), who had reportedly exorcised at least one woman at the communion rail (Hoyt, 1978), also was fiercely anti-Semitic and blamed the Jewish community in Russia for instigating the pogroms they suffered. He was also a strong supporter of the Tsar (Webb, 1976).

Unfortunately, in many places it appears that the ancient approach of beating a person believed to be possessed in order to make the demon leave continues to be standard practice (Taylor, 2007). The website http://whatstheharm.net/exorcisms.htm claims that they have evidence of 1,089 people who were harmed by exorcisms, a fact which must be looked at honestly if anyone is to engage in exorcisms or advocate for their relevance.

In a report by the BBC (2006), the debate about injuries during exorcisms quickly becomes multilayered. The reporting was initiated when the Metropolitan Police released a report which indicated the abuse of African immigrant children in the UK was widespread and connected with churches that believed in witchcraft and possession. These churches were predominantly immigrant churches. A later report, commissioned by the UK government and entitled "Child Abuse Linked to Accusations of Possession and Witchcraft" did indicate 74 cases of abuse over a 5-year period, a number that all agreed was too high but which was dramatically lower than the original suggestion in the Police report. Other suggestions in the Metropolitan report included accusations about children being sacrificed, a claim which was found to have no evidence and which is very similar to earlier claims about SRA (John, 2005) and multiple other communities as mentioned earlier in this text. The very legitimate concern about the health and wellbeing of children must also be tempered by the tendency to become suspicious of outrageous accusations, especially regarding groups that can be easily demonized, such as immigrant communities.

Sherwood (2017), a British journalist, covered a recent report about the frequency of exorcisms in the UK for the left-leaning paper *The Guardian*. The report, written by Ryan (2017) for a Christian think tank *The Theos,* does not dispute the possibility of demonic possession nor does it condemn exorcisms but rather worries that people may avoid proper mental health care, such as medication, in favor of exorcisms, which one psychiatrist is quoted in the article as stating would constitute "spiritual abuse" (Ryan, 2017, p. 24). That argument seems nuanced and understanding, which is reflected in the body of the article by Sherwood (2017). However, the headline to the article, "'Spiritual abuse': Christian think tank warns of sharp rise in UK exorcisms", seems to suggest it is the exorcism itself which is inherently abusive, an argument not made by Ryan (2017). It is also interesting to note that Sherwood (2017) only looks within the article to the formal Church of England for clarification on the issue outside of the cited paper by Ryan (2017), even though both the article and the paper discuss how much of the practice of exorcism is done by immigrant communities as well as other Pentecostal church communities.

Perceived Advantages to Exorcism

As a cultural phenomenon, demonic possession can be socially advantageous. African practices of exorcism continue to be widely practiced, although not among all tribes. Linde (2001), in a memoir of a year of mental health work in Zimbabwe, notes how some tribes emphasize possession and exorcism while others accept Western modalities or have alternative approaches to treatment.

Exorcism itself can mean very different things. Kugel (2013), in quoting the British anthropologist Godfrey Lienhardt, who worked with the Dinka people of southern Sudan, described a man who had been imprisoned in Khartoum and so named his son Khartoum. This was done to turn around harmful influences that the experience might have. Kigel claims: "The act is an act of exorcism, but the exorcism of what, for us, would be memories of experiences" (2013, p. 76). Scull (2015) notes how Yoruba rituals of healing in Nigeria often include the rauvolfia plant (Indian snakeroot), an alkaloid which has antipsychotic properties and had briefly been synthesized as reserpine, a pharmaceutical antipsychotic. The plant has also been used in Aryuvadic medicine in India.

Kiely and McKenna (2007) and McAll (1981) document exorcisms in England, Scotland, and Northern Ireland, and seem to include a specific focus on ghosts. McAll (1981) claims that possession may occur due to family dynamics, although it is clear here he means that the dead are somehow taking possession of the living in order to complete some unfinished work. While not explicitly cited, it seems likely that they are in the intellectual company of the Anglican Canon John D. Pearce-Higgins. He publicly differed from the promotion of the traditional understanding of the rite as an exorcism of demonic forces (Hoyt, 1978) and instead encouraged the belief that possession, as well as most hauntings, is the result of deceased persons who need guidance into the next phase of their journey as they have forgotten or refused to believe the fact that they have died. He refers to his practice as "persuasion exorcism" (Guiley, 2009, p. 79). He will often be accompanied by a medium, which is a practice most other Christian exorcists would frown upon, given the historic criticism of Spiritualism from traditionalist Christians (Hoyt, 1978).

Among some contemporary Pentecostals and evangelicals in America, deliverance is seen as a rite of passage (Cuneo, 2001; see also Cox, 1995), an interesting phenomenon in a tradition that has moved away from the Rite of Confirmation to indicate the transition into adulthood. Baglio (2009) cites the Association of Italian Catholic Psychiatrists and Psychologists that suggests more than half a million Italians see an exorcist yearly. Wilkinson (2007) writes as an American reporter while living in Rome. The book includes a long section on Fr. Amorth, who is one of the most famous Catholic exorcists. Wilkinson (2007) points out that the American edition to Amorth's (1999) memoir contains one of the oddest known forwards, penned by a Jesuit priest who is also a psychologist, Fr. Groeschel (1999). In it, he admits that he initially turned down the offer to write the forward. Even now, he is unable to write as a mental health professional; rather he is writing this as a priest who has reservations about the book.

In his practice, Fr. Amorth (1990, 1999) will ask if a possibly possessed person has consulted a doctor or a mental health professional, but then does not require such a differential diagnosis if they had not been seen by a mental health provider (Wilkinson, 2007), even performing the exorcism over the phone or after receiving an email (Guiley, 2009). Furthermore, he appears to believe that the exorcism itself is a form of differential diagnosis, a view which is controversial among exorcists (Wilkinson, 2007).

In another interview, this time with Monsignor Andrea Gemma, Wilkinson (2007) addresses the similarity of exorcism to therapy; "So, finding someone who listens and prays is important, even psychologically. Sometimes just the fact of being listened to, or being invited into prayer and into a relationship of trust, this is a great remedy for those who are suffering" (p. 83). Such a pastoral approach might suggest that a person like Monsignor Gemma would be an ally with mental health practitioners. Unfortunately, this does not seem to be the case. He has criticized the updated Catholic rite from 1999, which requires a medical evaluation, claiming that the medicine of prayer and exorcism is good "for every illness" (p. 84).

Levi-Strauss (1967), in contrasting the autobiography of a native shaman with contemporary practice (which in his day was still predominantly psychoanalytic), writes, "At any rate, it seems probable that medicine men, like their civilized colleagues, cure at least some of the cases treated and without this relative success magical practices could not have been so widely diffused in time and space" (p. 36). Torrey (1986) finds great similarity between shamanism (which he calls "witch doctoring") and modern mental health therapy. The contemporary psychotherapist Kottler (2003) also connects the effectiveness of therapy with the practice of shamanism and cites the work of Keeney (1996, 2003) as an example of other practitioners with similar leanings. Kottler (2003) shared in the text that he keeps soil he has received from an Incan traditional healer on his desk as a physical and visual reminder of those connections; however, he does look askance at the practice of exorcism. Al-Habeeb (2003), in researching faith healers in Saudi Arabia, documented their reports of high success rates but notes that differential diagnosis by individual healers, even for culturally understood ailments, varied widely. However, it is worth noting that such extremes are also found in Western therapeutic practice.

Women and Possession

Among members of the Zar tradition in Egypt, Ethiopia, and Sudan, it has been documented that women and effeminate men are those who tend to be possessed by outside (evil) spirits, only then to be exorcised by folk healers in a trance (Markis, 2000). Sawgi (2015) claims that a parallel male ritual in places such as Sudan is the trance dance used within Sufi Islam. The popularity of Zar has increased with the rise of fundamentalist understandings of Islam. An interpretation of this phenomenon is that Zar is a form of female protest and/or individual meaning-making against the rigid boundaries of a fundamentalist worldview, a role that Sufism also can play (see Armstrong, 2002). However, Zar practice also allows the patriarchal theological power structures to remain unchallenged directly (Wood, 2015b). Messing (1967) documents negative reasons for Zar possession, such as depression, addiction, and epilepsy.

Hoyt (1978) documents how the actual Zar exorcism varies; this is partially dependent upon the amount the family can pay the *shechah,* or exorcist. Messing (1967) notes a financial obligation, with the now exorcised person being expected to make lifelong donations to the Zar society. The Zar healer is a person who has experienced Zar possession and been able to integrate that aspect into their sense of self, a role that is similar to a sponsor found in 12 Step Recovery (Alcoholic Anonymous, 1981) as well as the notion of peer support specialists (Substance Abuse and Mental Health Services Administration, 2015).

Ecstatic dance, an animal sacrifice, the questioning of the Zar spirit (either in vernacular speech or in a special form of communication known only to the *shechah*), and then deliverance into an object in an alley or a bush are all included as possible in the rites (Markis, 2000; Hoyt, 1978). Some Zar possessed women replicate European modes of behavior or act excessively sexual (Wood, 2015b). The ability of a more powerful spirit to possess and drive out the lesser spirit, as well as the group music that is a part of the Zar rituals, is commented on by Eneborg (2015). Wood (2015b) notes how it is common for women who are undergoing a life transition, such as divorce, marriage, child birth, or the loss of a child, to become possessed by a Zar spirit. Schmidt (2015b) notes that in early studies of some Brazilian practices such as Candomblé, the rites were made up of women and effeminate men but that the movement has gained significant mainstream acceptance. Messing (1967) further notes the popularity of Zar among minority groups in Ethiopia, including Sudanese immigrants.

Wilkinson (2007) attempts to address why women throughout various cultures seem more likely to be possessed than men. For the traditionalists, women are seen as more open to temptation (see 1 Timothy 2:13-14). There is also a long history of mythological fear of women (Campbell, 1979). A medical belief in hysteria, which was believed to originate in the uterus, goes back to the Greeks (Porter, 2002). Demos (2008) notes that while men are sometimes implicated in the witch trials of the Middle Ages, it was mostly women who were accused of engaging in illicit connections to an always male Devil or devils. Russell (1972) points to the tendency of viewing women as witches, which begins to be common in the fifteenth century, until it became accepted that a witch was necessarily a woman. One aspect was the tendency of women to deal with herbs, cooking, birth, and other aspects tied to witchcraft, not only in Europe but in many parts of the world. The other aspect was the social change originating the courtly love tradition, which understood women to be not something less than a person but rather a more spiritual, pure, and delicate creature, susceptible and thus needing the protection of the brave knight. This tendency includes Hinduism, which can include female oracles of certain deities (Fibiger, 2015). Demos (2008) argues that there is an archetypical imaging at work here and points to the near universality of witch accusations well beyond Europe, this continues into the modern day. For Demos (2008), the female witch is the ultimate "Bad Mother" who brings destruction instead of new life, thus connecting to male anxiety about female fertility (p. 42).

Werse (2015a) cites the interesting case of the French woman Marthe Brossier (b. 1573). Her family was facing declining prospects, and she was not only unable to secure a marriage proposal, she was also declined by a nearby convent due to her father's inability to pay the customary contribution. She attempted to flee the area dressed as a man but was discovered and returned in shame to her home. By 1598, three years after several witches were executed in her hometown, she began to manifest symptoms of possession. During public exorcisms, in the voice of the demons, she denounced the recently legalized Protestant Huguenots. She did so both while she was in France and while she toured in Rome. The family was able to make significant sums from donations at these traveling exorcisms. Marthe also claimed a neighbor's family, particularly an older female, was behind this bewitchment The neighbor, Anne Chevreau (Guiley, 2009), made a detailed defense that is preserved in the records. Brossier was discovered as a fraud when she responded to Latin "prayers" that were in fact lines from Virgil, as well as recoiling from holy water that was unblessed. Chevreau claimed that Brossier was not ill-intentioned but was suffering from her shame and was manipulated by those around her.

Hoyt (1978) cites the work of Stanley and Ruth Freed (1976), anthropologists who studied possession in northern India soon after liberation from England. The Freeds document a young, newly married female possessed by the spirit of her friend who had died from suicide. The exorcism was successful, but when interviewed by the Freeds the young girl, named Daya in the text, admitted that the friend had committed suicide due to an unplanned premarital pregnancy and that Daya was very uncomfortable with her sexual relationship with her husband.

For Chaudhuri (2012), in a study of contemporary women working in tea plantations in India, women are targeted because they are occupants of lower status in society. Therefore, blame can be placed upon them without a chance of recourse, feeding into existing belief systems that only women are witches. Hoyt (1978) documents a case in Vienna in 1583 when a Jesuit priest spent 8 weeks exorcising a young woman whose symptoms consisted of severe menstrual cramping. Eventually her grandmother was tortured until confessing she was the source of the possession and was burned as a witch.

Oesterreich (1930) has pointed out the distinction within medieval thought separating witches from those possessed; witches would have at least some degree of sexual enjoyment in their connection with the devil, whereas those possessed experienced their state as always unpleasant and they entered into the state against their will (see also Stephens, 2002). Women have long had a tendency to be pathologized by authorities, be they religious or psychological (Clinebell, 1976). Treating women for hysteria was one of the main focuses of Freud, and women continue to be diagnosed with mental health issues at a higher rate than men (Ehrenrich, 2009), although it is also noted that women attend therapy at a higher rate than men. Some of the symptoms of hysteria are currently known as either Somatization disorder, that is multiple diffuse physical symptoms, or as Conversion disorder, which has a more limited and specific physical manifestation, such as a loss of sight (APA, 2013). The APA (2013) as well as all literature on the subject, note that Dissociative disorders, Borderline Personality Disorder, as well as Conversion and Somatization disorder, occur substantially more often in women than in men.

Amorth (1990, 1999) posits that women are more likely to be spiritually attuned and are thus more likely to see a priest if in trouble, which Baglio (2009) agrees with. Both Amorth (1990, 1999) and Baglio (2009) argue that women are also more likely to consult with the occult (see also Wilkinson, 2007). In Amorth's practice, he sees women three times more often than men (1990, 1999). This theory has an interesting parallel among some cognitive theorists who claim that women are more involved in religious activity due to a higher level of empathy (Schmidt, 2015b).

Wilkinson (2007) features several contemporary Italian women who regularly undergo exorcisms. One woman, Caterina, a professional dancer and dance instructor, had undergone psychological evaluation before seeing a Catholic exorcist. She was deemed to be schizophrenic with dissociative and anxious symptoms, a diagnosis which she dismisses. She tends to blame every bad event in her life on the devil, from her house burning down to a bumped knee, a tendency to avoid responsibility that Wilkinson finds common among those who seek out an exorcism (see also Chapter 9 with the interview with Fr. Tom, 2015). Francesca, another case study in Wilkinson (2007), is a doctor who specializes in urology. She suddenly began to have paralysis in different parts of her body, migraines, and hemorrhaging. Eventually, she had to stop her medical training because she felt that another power was moving her hands. She attributes her symptoms to a curse cast upon her by a rival for her fiancé's attention, a woman who ended up marrying him. Francesca sought out a number of medical opinions, including a psychiatrist, before being treated by Bishop Milingo, a controversial Catholic exorcist from Africa who lived at the time in Italy. The text is unclear about the outcome of the exorcisms.

Brotherton (2015) writes about proportionality bias, which means that we tend to attribute small consequences to small actions and vice versa. An example cited in the text is that when a person is attempting to roll a small number on a die, they will roll gently; in an attempt to get a large number, the same person will roll with force. This of course has no effect on the number that will be on the die. Brotherton states, "Likewise, when we're faced with a personal tragedy it can be tempting to think that it is part of some divine plan, or maybe the work of the Devil" (p. 211). This does not mean that such a belief is absurd, after all Brotherton claims to roll a die in the same way we all do. Rather, it is that much more important for a clinician or pastoral provider to help a patient acknowledge their own role and the origin of their suffering to help them bring about healing.

Contemporary Catholic Exorcisms

Baglio (2009) follows a Catholic priest in Rome, Fr. Thomas, an American who is undergoing training to become an exorcist. This book became the basis for the film *The Rite* (Flynn & Håfström, 2011). The movie was introduced in a film fest by the Catholic exorcist Fr. Gabriele Amorth (Laycock, 2015b). Burke (2011) notes that since returning to the States, Fr.

Thomas has exorcised 5 people in five years. Four of them stopped due to lack of progress. He is contacted by 40 people per month who are interested in possible exorcism, for which he requires a mental health consultation before proceeding. Both Baglio (2009) and Burke (2011) note the increased prevalence of outside consultation between priests and mental health professionals in America as opposed to Italy, which may be due to the increased social acceptance of mental health needs in the US, or the higher likelihood of legal consequences if outside consultation is not attempted.

Fr. Patella (2012), in writing about the intersection between mental health practice and exorcism, notes that with personality disorders like Borderline Personality Disorder (BPD) a person can tend toward obsessive thoughts, a characteristic of demonic oppression if not possession. It is interesting to note that he does not include Obsessive Compulsive Disorder or Obsessive Compulsive Personality Disorder as well in his description. The inclusion of BPD is interesting, as Dziegielewski (2010) has noted the tendency for BPD to be a more common diagnosis among female clients, and Kutchins and Kirk (2003) have noted that BPD tends to be a diagnosis given that demonizes the patient, especially if the patient is difficult or noncompliant.

Contemporary Catholic understanding of demonic influence stretches in a continuum from the ordinary to the extraordinary. Ordinary demonic influence would include pain that has no physical origin to obsessive thoughts. Oppression can include torments from demons and has been a common theme in hagiographies of saints. Subjugation is when a person is possessed, whereas infestation is when an object or space is possessed (Phillips, 2015b).

Zoja (1989) has written that one ongoing dynamic within contemporary society is an inability to deal with death. That inability is channeled into the subsequent rise in addictions as a personal form of death. For Catholics, Pope John Paul II was famous for critiquing contemporary society as a culture of death (1995), a stance which was rather broad in the encyclical in which it appears, but which quickly became interpreted as a statement solely on abortion and euthanasia, with the other listed social ills in the text (for example, poverty) largely ignored. If both writers are correct, then there appears to be a tension within the culture that both promotes a culture of death and also denies death. For Taylor (2007), a focus upon death is witnessed not only in Jungian and Catholic thought, but also in the anti-humanistic tendencies of Nietzsche and his intellectual decedents. While neither Zoja (1989) nor Pope John Paul II (1995) discuss the subsequent rise in the fascination with the occult in either text, Pope John Paul II promoted exorcisms strongly throughout his papacy (Baglio, 2009; Wilkinson, 2007).

Zoja (1989) writes that the resurgence in formerly dismissed or discredited rituals (he cites circumcision and New Age practices) shows the deep hunger in the contemporary person for a connection to ancient rites.

The Catholic focus on the demonic has continued, including by the recent Pontiff, Pope Francis I (Helmuth, 2014). In this article, the author interviews another journalist who witnessed an exorcism of an Italian woman by a priest connected with Fr. Amorth. It is of interest that in the lead up to the interview, there is a story shared about another Catholic priest/exorcist, Fr. Cesar Truqui, who attempted to silently pray for a lesbian woman whom he saw on a plane, until she threw chocolates at him and growled. The suspicious reader is left to suspect that Fr. Truqui may have been less than pastoral in his manner, especially given that her sexual orientation appears to be otherwise unconnected to the story.

The Exorcist in the 21st Century

In the documentary film *The Exorcist in the 21st Century* (Falsh & Akselsen, 2013), a number of religious exorcists are interviewed, including the Catholic Fr. Jose Antonio Fortea, the only exorcist in Spain and a prolific author, although almost all of his works are in Spanish. He is shown presiding over a mass in Bogota where he is treated almost like a rock star, mobbed by people after the conclusion of the service. He is then shown into a back room, filled with neatly aligned rows of people that he says prayers over as they are "slain by the spirit" (falling backward into the arms of attendants, a common experience among Charismatics and Pentecostals).

All, that is, except Constanza, a Columbian woman who believes she is possessed. Fr. Fortea cannot exorcise her, as he does not have dispensation to perform full blown exorcisms in that diocese. Interestingly enough, he does not refer her to another exorcist but rather encourages her to join a prayer group, a very pastoral answer. Thankfully, Constanza has received mental health care, as she admits to suicidal ideation as well as numerous life stressors as precursors to her possession state, including the loss of her job, health issues, the death of her mother, and a crisis in her marriage. Her psychiatrist, who is interviewed, does not attribute her symptoms to supernatural causes but does understand that she and her family do. She was diagnosed with major depressive disorder and placed on anti-depressants for a period of three years, but her attendance at therapy appears to have ended rather early. She is shown having clear explosive outbursts that appear to be in the voice of an alter. She does attend deliverance prayers, but complains they are always in a group. She desires a one-on-one exorcism, and ends up traveling from Columbia to Lima, Peru, for an exorcism performed by a minister in a different denomination, the Holy Catholic Apostolic Renovated Church of Peru (a small denomination that is structured like Catholicism but is more fundamentalist Protestant in theology, with such beliefs as the imminent second coming of God, and no theological schooling for pastors).

Fr. Jose Antonio Fortea is quoted in the movie strongly arguing against modern critical readings of the Bible (for example, historical criticism, which has been officially allowed by the Vatican as a legitimate tool) and instead claims the Bible itself must be read word for word literally, a claim which is itself outside the realm of official Catholic teaching but is common among Christian fundamentalism. This is immediately followed by a critique of the scientific claims of modernity. He claims the success of the film *The Exorcist* (Blatty & Frieden, 1973) was due directly to the will of God. Given the inherent short time, highly edited and de-contextualized nature of film documentaries, I hesitate to say this is a complete or necessarily accurate portrayal of Fr. Fortea, especially as I have not read his published writings given my Spanish is quite poor. However, if the interview is an accurate presentation of him, he appears to be rather fundamentalist in his understanding of his faith.

The film includes other interviews of priests, including the Catholic bishop of Norway, Fr. Bernt Eidsvig, who holds strictly to the need for a full mental health evaluation before referral for exorcisms to be performed. He estimated that about 15 Norwegians a year request the rite and one or two are granted it. The Rite is performed by an exorcist from another country as Norway has no exorcist among Catholic clergy. Fr. Amorth is also interviewed in the film and goes on a rather long rant about how exorcists are not respected by other priests within the church (see also Cumo, 2015). Interestingly, due to his rather high profile, he has a very small role in the documentary. The film shows a plurality of views within Catholicism on the role of the devil and the place of exorcism. It appears likely that such a continuum of belief will continue, as the Roman Catholic Church tends toward an allowance of broad disagreement in certain areas (as shown by the plethora of religious orders), but a very clear demarcation of other beliefs and practices, such of sexual morality.

SECTION 2

CHAPTER FOUR

MULTIPLE PERSONALITY DISORDER/ DISSOCIATIVE IDENTITY DISORDER

Early Descriptions

Goodman (1988b) notes that descriptions of multiple personalities did not appear in Europe until the eighteenth century, when the Age of Enlightenment began the separation of religious belief from other aspects of human life. She does not mention Foucault's (1961, trans. 1973; 1966, trans. 1973) analysis of that era, including the institutionalization and penalization of persons with mental health issues. Crabtree (1997a) claims the first documented case of multiple personalities was done in 1816 by Dr. S. L. Mitchill, a physician in New York City who was working with a patient named Mary Reynolds.

It may be argued that the famous novella of Robert Louis Stevenson, *The Strange Case of Dr. Jekyll and Mr. Hyde* (1886, 2003), in which the consumption of a liquid changes the good Dr. Jekyll into a murderous villain, is a story of multiple personality, although it may also be read as an allegory on such wide ranging themes as substance abuse, closeted homosexuality, and even the torn allegiance of the Scottish people (Nabokov, 2003; *The Guardian*, 2008). Jung (1968) has written that the book itself came to the author initially in a dream. The text has had well over a hundred film, theatre, and TV adaptations (Egan, 2013) and has influenced numerous other authors, including Eco (2011), whose novel includes a person unaware of the murderous acts of their alter. As an interesting aside, Crabtree (1997a) has documented how Stevenson attributed his creative talents to possession by "little people" or "brownies" inside of himself.

Moyano, et al. (2001) document how dissociation, understood as a form of hysterical neurosis, was a common diagnosis from 1890 until 1910 among various mental health professionals. Nakatani (2000) attributes some of this understanding to the influence of Pierre Janet (1859-1947), a man whose writings are not much translated into English but who had tremendous influence on not only Freud but all of depth psychology, the theoretical force of the time. For example, Crabtree (1997a) cites a case which Janet published in 1890, where Janet suggests a second personality to a patient who then names it herself, all during a course of hypnosis. However, after 1910, the diagnosis tended to disappear until it was rediscovered by those who were working with patients with trauma histories.

Contemporary understanding of Multiple Personality

In more modern times, multiple personalities became well known in part due to the popularity of a novel by Shirley Jackson, *The Bird's Nest* (1954), as well as a case study by Thigpen and Cleckley (1957), *The Three Faces of Eve*, which was then made into a movie also released in 1957 (Johnson & Johnson). In that case, the woman in question continued to separate into alters until later therapy by other providers, who were successful in integrating her personalities into one. She documented the unsuccessful (but popularized) therapy and the later success in integrating her alters in a memoir entitled *I'm Eve* (Siezmore & Pittillo, 1977; see also Crabtree, 1997a). There was a popular novelization of another case, *Sybil* by Flora Rheta Schreiber (1973), which describes the therapy of a young woman with multiple personalities by psychiatrist Dr. Cornelia Wilbur, which was also made into a TV film in 1976 (Babbin & Petrie), with another version done in 2007 (Mahoney & Sargent).

Multiple personality disorder was first included in the DSM-III (American Psychiatric Association, 1980); previously it was seen as a type of conversion disorder, but the diagnosis was understood as a type of hysteria. It was first involved in a court case involving a man named Billy Milligan, who was charged with multiple rapes. His case revolved around having over 20 distinct personalities, although the actual assaults were supposedly committed by two alters, a Yugoslavian communist Ragan, and a lesbian named Adalana. Billy was found not guilty due to insanity by a court in Ohio (Keyes, 1981) and recently passed away from cancer (Woods, 2014). As a result of his trial, Ohio has made it harder to use insanity as a defense, due in part to widespread doubt about the validity of his illness, although there are others who have no doubt he was very ill (see Crabtree, 1997a).

There was a significant uptick in diagnoses of multiple personality disorder in the 1970s, notably before it became formalized as a recognized disorder in the DSM. Numerous writers of that time note the increase of this phenomenon without any explanation as to why (e.g.; Allison & Schwartz, 1980; Beal, 1978; Brendsma & Ludwig, 1974; Putman, 1985). Goodman

(1988b) claims that the popularity of new religious expressions and drug experimentation allowed people to access ASCs which they were then unable to explain. However, she does not offer any evidence to indicate that people experiencing MPE/DID had a history with drugs use or New Age participation. Nakatani (2000) attributes the increase in MPE to a variety of factors: feminism's focus on the all too common experiences of childhood abuse, the very high prevalence of PTSD among Vietnam veterans and concentration camp survivors, as well as the media's repeated use of MPE as a theme, creating an echo chamber effect. A character with MPE is treated in the bestselling Yalom text *Love's Executioner* (1989), which consists of fictionalized case studies presumably from his own clinical practice.

It is worth noting that the diagnosis of MPE tends to be associated with patients who have a high risk of suicidality and high rates of childhood trauma. This is often sexual but can include other intended or unintended traumas, a trend also seen among patients with diagnoses of BPD, PTSD, and substance use disorders (Foote, et al., 2008). Among German patients hospitalized in a psychiatric setting, Gast, et al. (2001) found a clear statistical correlation between childhood trauma and rates of dissociative symptoms. Sar, Alioğlu, and Akyüz (2014) did a survey of Turkish women which indicates that, in a culture that embraces possession as a way of understanding psychic pain, the experiences of a traumatic past and PTSD symptoms are more likely to result in experiencing possession states. Ross (2011) compares patients' diagnoses with DID from the US and Canada with a general population (control) sample from Winnipeg as well as an outpatient mental health patient sample from China. In this study, ASCs such as trance, possession states, sleepwalking, and paranormal experiences are much higher among those with DID than in both the Chinese mental health patients and the general population Canadian group.

A memoir by a person with an MPE diagnosis was penned by Tayja Wiger (with Cynthia Bend, 1988). Wiger has a number of physical ailments, including cerebral palsy and blindness, as well as schizophrenia and substance use issues. Her upbringing was deeply traumatic, but she came to a sense of healing and meaning by embracing shamanism and becoming an ordained minister. Her memoir is rather scattered and difficult to follow (the text is a weaving of Wiger's therapeutic journals and extensive excerpts from scholarly and New Age writings), but her life story presents an example of how integrative approaches can be powerfully healing for patients.

The Change to Dissociative Identity Disorder

When the APA changed the diagnosis of MPD to Dissociative Identity Disorder in the DSM-IV (APA, 1994), Dr. Spiegel, one of the authors of the new text, was noted as saying that the reason for the change was that patients were not suffering from multiple personalities, rather they had less than one full personality (Loftus & Kitchum, 1994). Crabtree (1997a), Ofshe and Watters (1994), and Loftus and Ketcham (1994) argue instead that a multiple personality is created, in part, by the therapeutic alliance that forms between a suffering patient and a well-meaning but harm-causing clinician. One reason is the contagion found in group therapy among this population, a phenomenon also observed among the youth who engage in forms of self-mutilation such as cutting (Richardson & Surmitis, 2014).

As described in the revision to the 4th edition, known as the DSM-IV TR (APA, 2000), a person who exhibits the symptoms of DID but whose alters are demons or other spirits of the dead would have been best diagnosed as having Dissociative Disorder Not Otherwise Specified (or NOS). Two other diagnoses mentioned for further research in the manual were Dissociative Trance Disorder (DTD) and Possession Trance Disorder (PTD). In a study of persons in Uganda who were experiencing what they believed to be possession symptoms, Van Duijl, Kleijn, and de Jong (2013) found no discernable difference between DTD and PTD. In another study of 10 persons who reported possession and were in in-patient hospital settings, Ferracuti, Sacco, and Lazzari (1996) found a similarity between DTP and PTD, suggested a dissociative continuum in actual experience. During, et al. (2011) reviewed the existing medical literature of DTD up to that time. The findings were that the vast majority (60%) of the 402 people who had been documented had possession symptoms, one in 5 had amnesia, 56% reported hallucinations, and somatic complaints were found in 34%. There was no single explanation in the literature for the cause of the possession event.

Lewis (2015b) documents, although without a citation, the formation of a committee of mental health practitioners and anthropologists that worked for a decade inside the APA on helping to revise the DSM to be sensitive to trance and other dissociative symptoms (albeit with real resistance from some). As mentioned above, in the newest edition of the DSM (APA, 2013), DID diagnosis is now explicitly open to possession as a manifestation of alters, a change that was earlier reflected in some of the literature (i.e. Spiegel, et al., 2011). However it is labeled, the symptoms are similar in the formal diagnosis known alternatively as MPD/DPD-NOS/DTP/PTD/DID and possession as described in the text, including facial contortions, muscle tension, as well as the experience of an alien entity inhabiting the psyche (Goodman, 1988b).

In the new DSM diagnosis (APA, 2013), there is a dissociative subtype of PTSD, a change which has international evidence (Stein, et al. 2013). At present, this subtype does not include any reference to possession states, although future editions might want to examine this as a possible diagnostic subtype. Spiegel, et al. (2013) argued for including conversion disorder, in with dissociative disorders, although that did not happen in the DSM-5 (APA, 2013).

It is widely believed that the dissociation is often, but not exclusively, due to trauma or other overwhelming experiences (Spiegel, et al., 2011). Cardena and Gleaves (2007) state that the trauma is usually childhood abuse, although it can include other significant events. From an international perspective, Van Duijl, Kleijn, and de Jong (2013), note a higher rate of past traumatic events among those with dissociation/possession symptoms (as diagnosed by traditional healers) when compared to a control group in Uganda. It is worth noting in this study that the identified traumas include many that occurred in adulthood, which is likely due to the instability in both the country and that region during the lifetime of those studied. It is also interesting that those in this study who had dissociation/possession symptoms and traumatic experiences did not see a connection between the two.

The Iatrogenic Controversy

In one of the most famous of cases involving a person with multiples, Eve Lancaster (1958) states that at the end of her treatment with Drs. Thigpen and Cleckey, she went from three alters to sixteen. In another famous case, Dr. Herbert Spiegel had seen the original client who was the basis of "Sybil" several times and disagreed with Dr. Wilbur, claiming that "Sybil" was being manipulated for the sake of fame and financial gain (Borch-Jacobsen, 1997; see also Rieber, 1998). The name for this phenomenon is iatrogenic. Tammy Bell (1990) uses the classic example of an iatrogenic disease when she describes a surgeon who doesn't wash between operations, thereby causing infection among those who were already sick (see also Illich, 1982). This may happen by intention or by accident. Kottler (2003) claims that those who point out iatrogenic causes tend to be poorly received by their colleagues, which is perhaps not surprising.

In an article by Spanos, et al. (1991), the authors describe a study in which participants were encouraged to remember a past life under hypnosis.

Those participants who were given suggestions of abuse in the past life created memories of such abuse. For Loftus and Kitchum (1994), who are writing about false repressed memories, this is evidence of the power of the therapist for suggestion. Loftus and Kitchum (1994) argue that it is normal for people who are hypnotized to create memories on their own or be highly suggestible to the therapist's beliefs or desires. Wilkinson (2007) stated, "A good hypnotist can make a patient bark like a dog. An exorcist, less explicitly and unintentionally, can make a patient talk like the devil" (p. 151). Ganaway (1989) has written that MPD/DID is a created diagnosis, exacerbated by the clinical use of hypnosis. Graves (1988) argues strongly that the MPD diagnosis cannot be iatrogenic and then claims that those who doubt such a diagnosis are engaging in a counter-transference reaction to the nightmarish stories of childhood abuse. McHugh (1995) has argued that MPD is always iatrogenic, and therapeutic goals would include ignoring any "alters" so that the personality can do their own work. This is in marked contrast to the prevailing therapeutic approach, which is to engage directly with the alters, presuming that they have therapeutic information to share. The therapist does attempt to decrease the number of alters and thus integrate their multiplicity of voices into a coherent personality, but one who is better able to negotiate the world (Jongsma & Peterson, 2006; Spiegel, et al., 2011).

For Boysen and Van Bergen (2013), the very validity of the MPE/DID diagnosis is in question. The authors examined the published scholarly research on DID from 2000 to 2010 and discovered that the diagnosis of MPE/DID was practically non-existent outside a limited number of clinicians in a few countries. Furthermore, DID symptoms could be reproduced in laboratory settings by otherwise non-symptomatic actors and be indistinguishable from those with the formal diagnosis. One is left to wonder if the same result could have been produced by actors playing psychotic, anxious, or depressed patients as well, which is not mentioned in the paper.

Foote, et al. (2008) note that in a small study of 231 patients in an inner-city psychiatric hospital, many met the diagnostic criteria of MPE/DID without having the diagnoses. The authors theorize that among certain populations (e.g. people living in high poverty, those with a history of childhood trauma, and survivors of warfare), DID symptoms might be more prevalent than previously thought or currently diagnosed. Cross-culturally, Ginzburg, et al. (2010) looked at DID diagnoses in Israel and found that one-half of mental health practitioners in the country did not believe in the validity of the diagnoses. However, the authors note that about one-quarter of the surveyed residents in a psychiatric hospital (82 patients in total) met the diagnostic criteria for DID. There is evidence for the similarity in traits among patients with DID across cultures, for example, Sar, Yargic and Tutkun's (1996) survey of Turkish sufferers.

Personally, I know of one case of self-diagnosed DID/MPD being an iatrogenic disease. The person took an online personality profile through Facebook (obviously, this was not a formal assessment like the MMPI). The profile suggested that their other personality was a dog. From that point on, this person wore a dog collar and would act out certain canine characteristics. This person did not have the formal DID diagnosis, but did have many other diagnoses, including low intellectual functioning. It is clear that while this profile gave the person permission to act out in one way, another suggestion would have given permission for other behaviors, perhaps even demonic possession.

Diagnostic Challenges

Changes to the DSM due to concerns about implications of the diagnosis, as well as an attempt to better understand and classify the suffering of the patient, are nothing new. Perhaps a famous example is the hysterical neurosis diagnosis which was given primarily to women in the late 1800s and into the early part of the 1900s, and which constituted that majority of Freud and Jung's case load (Scull, 2012). Classification first appeared in the DSM-II and was renamed histrionic personality disorder in the DSM-III. Bakkevig and Sigmund (2010) argue that this change was made in order to differentiate it from the negative implications of hysteria, which would include confusion with demonic possession. Those authors doubt the validity of the diagnosis of histrionic personality disorder.

In the DSM-5, it is only DID which allows for belief in an outside possession (APA, 2013). However, numerous other diagnoses manifest in ways that could be understood as being caused by outside forces. These can include histrionic personality disorder as well as schizophrenia and other types of psychosis.

CHAPTER FIVE

POST-MODERNITY AND RELIGION

Modernity has been defined, at least in the context of this text, as when a mechanical worldview becomes dominant. This results in a subsequent disenchantment of the world. There are contemporary writers who have questioned the assumptions that underline modernity. Collectively, this line of thinking is known as post-modernism, although thinkers and approaches differ widely, making post-modernism hard to define. Dating the origins of, or even clearly defining post-modernity itself, has proven to be incredibly difficult (Berger, 1997; Kung, 1987, trans. 1988). Harvey (1989) claims it was the disappointment of the perfectibility of the human condition in "death camps and death squads, its militarism and two world wars, its threat of nuclear annihilation and its experience of Hiroshima and Nagasaki" that signaled the beginning of post-modernity. White (2006) distinguishes post-modernity as a historical era defined by observable phenomena such as the digital revolution, post-colonial power, and new scientific discoveries that challenged previous understandings of the world, such as quantum mechanics.

Post-modernism reflects viewpoints and worldviews that tend to be discordant and contradictory, rejecting a synthesizing totality. Harvey (1989) cites as intellectual precursors the Dada artistic movement after World War I, the German philosopher Friedrich Nietzsche (1844-1900), and somewhat surprisingly, St. Augustine of Hippo (354-430). During modernity, many professional fields, including the field of psychology, were hostile to religious thought (Frankl, 1969, 1988). Marsden (1997) has shown how higher learning has actively discouraged religious concepts from being taken seriously, a situation that had been common among mental health providers (Ivey, D'Andrea & Ivey, 2012).

The psychologist Robert Coles, in a conversation with Krista Tippets, quoted Flannery O'Conner, "Mystery is a great embarrassment to the modern mind" (NPR, Tippet, 2016, n.p.). However, Moshe Halbertal (2012), an Israeli philosopher, has stated: "Post-modernism has been kind to all religions. Reason was dethroned; there's no larger narrative out there anymore" (p. 3). Kuhn (1962) argues that science tends to create dogmatic belief systems that eventually get challenged in intellectual revolutions, termed "paradigm shifts". It would appear that the arrival of post-modernity has included such a shift. Tippet (2012) notes that the current post-modern challenge is to be simultaneously pluralistic and yet remain grounded.

In writing about his experience as a Church of Jesus Christ of Latter Day Saints (Mormon) missionary in Guatemala, the presumably pseudonymous Jacob (2013) described being involved in several exorcisms with a local woman with the help of the local, native Mormon bishop. Jacob, who identified himself as a modernist and a believer in science while also a devout Mormon, identified the thinking of Ludwig Wittgenstein (1954) and his use of "language games" as a way of understanding the tension between science and religion. While Jacob at home follows a scientific worldview that would presume possession narratives to be grounded in mental health concerns, in Guatemala he will use the indigenous understanding that this woman's suffering is based on a world of spirits. (It should be noted that this is not what Wittgenstein (1954) had in mind, but it is closer to the later writer Lyotard (1997), who built upon language games in developing a theory of metanarratives, which is what Jacob is really referring to.)

Enchantment

Midelfort (2005) has argued that modernity stripped the world of its spiritual implications. Starr (1984) makes the claim that this process began with the Reformation, which replaced a saint-mediated world with a direct connection to the Divine. When modernity challenged the existence of God, the world was then stripped of all value except for the economic value. The task at hand is now to re-enchant the world; either through a rediscovery of past practices or a discovery of future approaches that allow for a plurality of visions (see also Berman, 1981; Griffin, 2000; McGrath, 2003). Morris (2011) claims that all societies refer to the disenchantment of the now and yearn for a re-enchantment of the future that deeply echoes the glories of a past golden age. If Morris is correct, the contemporary feelings of disenchantment are not symptomatic of post-modern angst but are rather a part of the human condition. Zoja (1989) also questions if it is possible to create rituals anew, as if out of whole cloth, as opposed to letting them manifest in organic ways. This seems especially important among those who have left traditional religious communities.

Literature has long been struggling with the disenchantment of the world. T. S. Eliot (1925/1991), wrote one of the most quoted poems of the 20th century, the "Hollow Men" soon after the end of the First World War, a war which revealed the utter brutality that lay under the notion of civilization. The poem is written from the voice of the scarecrow/effigy of Guy Fawkes which appears to be speaking from some type of hell (Elliot references Dante several times throughout the poem). The theme of burning/hell corresponds symbolically with the lighting of bonfires to burn the effigy of Fawkes. The poem opens with a line from Joseph Conrad's *Heart of Darkness* (1902/1990), which details not only the brutality of the Belgian colonization of the Congo, but also is a mytho-psychological journey into the darkness within the narrator. The poem, like much that involves an interest in possession, ends with the apocalyptic end of the world, "This is how the world ends, not with a cry but with a whimper" (p. 82). Death, damnation, destruction, and emptiness; for Eliot the world is filled with those who, if not possessed, are at least hollowed. Within the poem there is also the Christian hope that within one's hollow self, there remains the chance to be hallowed.

Social Power

Numerous thinkers of post-modernism, like Michel Foucault (1961, trans. 1973; 1966, trans. 1973), have argued that mental illness is always understood within a social system, a system that is very hard for a person within it to escape from or even at times identify. A parallel might be seen in Fox's (1967) study of Pueblo people in the American Southwest. Illness within that culture required seeking a cure from one of the secret cultic societies, which reinforces their social power for the entire community. However, this system of healing also helped to reintegrate persons once they were sick or bewitched, as the Pueblo people place great emphasis upon witches as a cause of sickness. The dark side of this is the witch-hunt to find the person responsible, who might be executed.

Modernity for Foucault has included the separation of the "mad" from the "sane". Included in that separation is an anxiety about proper levels of control for those who are mad, including their institutionalization. Porter (2002), while taking some issue with the degree in which Foucault (1961, trans. 1973; 1966, trans. 1973) makes the argument, in essence agrees with his assessment of the nature of modernity to pathologize and separate people who were once more fully integrated within their communities. Scull (2015) notes that Foucault has a tendency to misinterpret symbolism as historic fact, such as the recurrent image of a "ship of fools" as being in reality a medieval intervention for those who were suffering, when Scull points out it was a recurrent image and motif but not a physical reality.

Monk and colleagues (1997), in advocating for a post-modern approach to counseling, have written:

> For example, it is accepted that people of 'other' cultures can develop 'culture-bound syndromes' . . . [but] the possibility of culture-bound syndromes in dominant white, Western culture tends to be ignored or un-researched. It seems to be assumed that more 'developed' cultures do not engender or exhibit such conditions. (p. 132).

The failure to recognize culture-bound symptoms within dominate Western culture(s) appears to be changing, as seen in the debate about MPD (which was covered in the previous chapter), as well as self-cutting (Richardson & Surmitis, 2014). Using these categories, the diagnosis of MPD/DID can be both iatrogenic and helpful, as it explains the psychic pain the patient is experiencing. This appears to parallel the hysterical neurosis that Freud was seeing in his practice, a culturally shaped way of manifesting psychological distress (Ehrenrich, 2009).

Demonic possession can be seen as a symptom of a previous, backward world that is lacking in knowledge and sophistication. However, the continued presence of exorcisms, even among fully modern persons, might indicate that modern tendencies to separate and diagnose may be incomplete, as this may be the language the patient has in explaining their distress. Furthermore, the modern tendency to dismiss such a phenomenon (e.g. Shermer, 2003) can further isolate the already suffering person.

In writing about the post-modern challenge to religion, Hans Küng (1985, trans. 1986) states, "religion is not in need of a restoration (which would, in the final analysis, be doomed), but of transformation, pregnant with hope for the future" (p. 56). Schenk writes that with post-modernism, "(m)eaning flits about, eluding categories, and words cannot escape the relativization of quotation marks… understanding becomes unfixed, a matter of allusion, sand play, as interpretation caves in on itself" (Schenk, 2001 p. xi). Thus, in a post-modern world, ancient explanations resurface to explain some very contemporary worries.

The plurality of meanings that is common among post-modern thought allows for the mechanical approaches that modernity encourages (and many mental health practitioners ascribe to) while also understanding that belief systems can include such concepts as unwanted spirit possession. It is no longer a question of either/or, rather we have moved to a both/and approach. As such, while looking at the DID diagnostic criteria, the DSM-5 can be seen as a post-modern text, in that it allows for both the worldview of the patient and the clinician to exist simultaneously, even if they are in conflict. Further, when looking at treatment, the two can inform each other, as we will discuss in the last chapter.

CHAPTER SIX

SOCIAL DYNAMICS

Possession as protest

Winzeler (2012) claims that the two primary purposes of involuntary spirit possession are a personal response to trauma and as a socially acceptable protest. The first purpose fits with the dominant understanding by mental health providers and an earlier generation of anthropologists, such as in Spiro's (1967) anthropological study in Burma. This understanding also fits with the DSM-5 understanding of DID etiology (APA, 2013). The protest theory has been advanced by Lewis (1986/2003) and picked up by other contemporary anthropologists. Under the protest theory, the possessed individual is almost always a member of the poorer class, is usually a woman, and is reacting to oppression in one of the only socially acceptable ways available.

Lewis (1986/2003) further states that this protest dynamic is found almost exclusively when there is a complex religious dynamic involved, where one religion (usually a worldwide one) has taken a dominant role, leaving the local religion in a peripheral role. Although not cited directly, Vásquez (2015) presents an example with the Gnawa in Morocco, who are decedents of former slaves and practice a form of voluntary jinn possession in order to bring about healing. The ritual not only appears to invoke the pre-Islamic tradition of the Gnawa ancestors, but also appears to be a ritual acting out of their history of liberation from slavery, similar to the Jewish celebration of Passover.

To back up Lewis' argument (1986/2003), Winzeler (2012) cites the cases that he observed of young Malay women in the 1970s and 1980s. One reoccurring situation in traditional areas was that high schools, which had not previously accepted females, began to experience cases of group hysteria among the young woman who had recently enrolled. The women would have fits of laughing, crying, or screaming, and then would report seeing visions of spirits. The disruptions at the schools were only remedied by bringing in either a Muslim imam or a traditional healer, a *bomoh* (Winzeler, 2012). At the same time as this was occurring in traditional parts of Malaysia, in the more modern factories some women reported similar experiences (Ong, 1987). Ong sites the low wages and long hours, with little to no possible remedy, as contributing factors in these women's unknowing use of spirit possession as protest.

Hegeman (2013) points out three further examples of possession as protest: the Zar cult in Sudan, *ataque* in Puerto Rico, and trance dance in Bali. In all three, multiple reasons for the experience are explained, including an escape from unpleasant reality, an expression of unmet desires and needs, an ability to become who or what the external authority has denied, and finally a process of dealing with trauma. Jong and Ries (2013) argue, in studying a possession cult of Kiyang-yang in the Western African nation of Guinea, that disassociation allows a collective expression of distress as well as the personal and collective processing of trauma. Lloyd (2015b) examines Lewis' (1986/2003) theory, invoking the work of Gomm (1975) among the Digo people of Kenya. Gomm (1975) notes how Digo women have a status much like children within the society, but when possessed they can demand money for various needs. Possession often occurs on payday. Lloyd (2015b) notes how, contrary to Lewis (1986/2003), this dynamic reinforces the status quo, as no real change in financial status is accomplished.

While not mentioned in the literature, the case of Aleister Crowley (1875-1947) may be another example of possession, and in this case interest in the occult itself, as a form of protest. Raised in the very devout family of fundamentalist Plymouth Brethren in England, he quickly embraced his mother's claim that he was "The Beast" from the Biblical Book of Revelation and used it as a name for himself (Guiley, 2009). He spent his life engaging in various occult activities and was adept at alienating many. He is reported to have experienced demonic possession after his involvement in a ritual, and ended up dying as a result of his heroin addiction.

According to Davies (1995), possession states are always social. Greenblatt has stated that exorcism is a form of performance (1988). The exorcism performed at the Pentagon during the Vietnam War as part of the anti-war movement (McKannon, 2011) is one example, as is the Catholic Bishop of Springfield, Illinois' public exorcism after the state legalized same-sex marriage (Laycock, 2015). Levi-Strauss (1967) connects the public aspect of healing to the work of tribal shamans; those who are not viewed as successful within their society lose their roles as healers, thus creating environments that encourage the theatrical in the process.

The social element of possession states has also been connected with amnesia in individuals; in societies where possession states are believed to be connected with amnesia, the individual will experience a loss of memories; in societies where it is not connected, the individual will remember their experiences (Goodman, 1988b). The current DSM indicates the likelihood of amnesia for DID but does not require it for diagnosis (APA, 2013). These anthropological findings may also be found when there is social doubt in possession, but individual belief reinforced by a clinical or pastoral belief, a dynamic found in the contemporary American practices of Peck (2005). If an individual feels they are possessed and there is no validation from outside of their experiences, the situation has become pathologized.

Lowe (1972) has posited three categories of consciousness: institution, symbolic order, and perspective. Institution is the social order which, if it undergoes massive change in an individual's life, is seen as destabilizing. This results in an individual relying on their perspective to find or create a symbolic order. If no symbolic order can be discovered outside of the self, Lowe asserts that the individual, like the characters in Dostoyevsky's novel *The Devils* (sometimes translated as *The Possessed,* 1872, 2009), falls into nihilistic patterns of despair or destructive action. This struggle arises in an attempt to force order into the other two categories, institution and social order.

Russell (1971) makes the argument that massive social change has led to a widespread belief in possession and a fear of heresy, all occurring during the rise of Western European cities. Burke (2011) quotes Nancy Caciola, who states that possession is common when religious institutions face serious challenges. Cuneo (2001) has contextualized the rise of possession and exorcism among Catholics within a social environment that has minimized organized religion and within an institution that has weathered serious scandals, including child sex abuse. The role of the exorcist, however, puts the priest into a hero mold. The exorcist is supposed to be "humble, of blameless life, courageous and a man of scholarship and learning" (Hoyt, 1979, p. 34), in other words an ideal priest as opposed to a child abuser. Burke (2011) and Cuneo (2001) also note how belief in demonic possession tends to be connected to apocalyptic beliefs.

For Mischel and Mischel (1958), possession not only elevates the status of the individual and allows for cathartic actions that are otherwise forbidden, the phenomenon also frees up the person from normal drudgery and allows (if the possessing spirit is other-gendered) a change in rigid gender roles. Prince (1966), after citing the previous findings, argues that a further advantage is a tightening of the social structure, the possessed person can "act out" and the group tightens up.

Davies (1995) further points out that spirits have other perspectives; what they have to say is often deemed important, as in the case of oracles or shamanistic practices (see also DuBois, 2009). Note that this, at least in most Christian exorcisms, is often not extended to demonic possession, as the statements of the possessing demons are presumed to be untrustworthy (Amarth, 1999; Koningisor, 2011; Peck, 2005). One notable exception is the German woman Anneliese Michel (Goodman, 1988b; Kiely & McKenna, 2007), whose critical statements about Vatican II while undergoing exorcisms were read with great interest by some conservative members of the church. It seems likely that if the spirit/demon speaks in a way that is contrary to what the community and/or exorcist wants to hear, their statements can be quickly discredited. Within Islam, the tendency to question the possessing Jinn is more common, according to Eneborg (2015).

Davies (1995) has argued that possession is a coping mechanism, a technique that allows the possessed person to act out in ways that are otherwise forbidden. Thus, it is a social steam valve, a release for both an individual who can speak and act in otherwise taboo ways, and the collective which witnesses and affirms the performance, either by listening to the oracles from the spirits or attempting to exorcize the demons. This is at least one common interpretation of the common trance and possession in Balinese rituals. In this otherwise composed society, up to seven different types of possessed persons are allowed a great degree of emotional expression (Lewis, 2015a). It is worth noting that within Roman Catholicism, the exorcism should not be a public act (Hoyt, 1978), although a number of exorcists have written luridly of their ministry (e.g. Amorth, 1989; Martin, 1976), making the work itself public.

Possession is not without serious consequences, including possibly ostracism, beatings, and even death (Cuneo, 2001; Kiely & McKenna, 2007) and there are many unfortunate examples of people believed to be possessed who experience horrifying abuses. This is why it can be an action of last resort (Davies, 1995). However, depending on the society and the type of possessing spirit, the act of possession might elevate the status of the individual (Lewis, 1986/2003).

Lewis (1986/2003) identifies spirit possession within social power; those without power can use the out-of-time experience of possession for a variety of reasons, including: protest, attention, and stress release. This does not appear to be the case in some contemporary European societies, such as Ireland (Kiely & McKenna, 2007) and Italy (Baglio, 2009), where the society is more heterogenic. Spirit possession also has fewer social implications than claiming bewitchment, which in many cultures carries with it serious implications from possibly hostile neighbors (Russell, 1971; Stephens, 2002).

The possession as protest theme can also lead to armed rebellion, as has been cited in Chapter 1 in regards to the Lord's Resistance Army in Uganda within our own time (Sagert, 2015a). Another example historically was Hong Xiuquan (1814-1864) a Chinese man who, after failing the civil service exam, experienced a shaman-like vision during which he was told he was the brother of Jesus. He led forces in the Taiping rebellion against the existing Chinese ruling Qing dynasty from 1853 to 1864 and is widely credited with laying the groundwork for the Boxer Rebellion a generation later (Haar, 2015).

Possession as Role Play

Bourguignon (1976) has advanced the theory that possession is a form of role-play; that the person possessed has a degree of autonomy in the enacting of the possession. Other anthropologists like Herskovits (1971) have argued that their experiences of possessed people seem to indicate at least the belief within the possessed person that this is a real experience. Personally, I acted out a demonic possession performance while in Catholic high school. At a classmate's party several people stated they were bored, and I decided to pretend to be possessed by a demonic entity. It was entertaining until I was almost expelled from school for the stunt. Looking back on it, there was a level of adolescent protest against the school, but there was more of a sense of symbolic asserting of my-self, an act of differentiation. For me, I had no sense that the experience was real, a fact which was not true among some of my schoolmates.

In a study reported by Baglio (2009), done by an Italian psychiatrist, Dr. Guiliana Mazzoni, subjects were studied on how memory can help shape beliefs. Subjects were told to read articles about possession, then asked questions about their fears, which were interpreted as if they had somehow witnessed a possession or exorcism in the forgotten past. Finally, subjects were told to rate the possibility that they had somehow seen a possession in the past. It was shown in the study that up to 25% of subjects created a false belief/memory that they had seen a possession, particularly if the original articles were about their own culture. Baglio (2009) questions the connection between societal reinforcement and reports about supernatural behavior (e.g. levitation, vomiting strange objects) in exorcisms. Among objective observers (Cuneo, 20001; Midelfort, 2005; Wilkinson, 2007) and even some advocates like Peck (2005), there is a marked absence of these events, in spite of exorcists claiming that they are common (e.g. Amorth,

1999). This could lead skeptics to charge that the supposed supernatural phenomena as reported by exorcism advocates like Amorth (1999) may be due to the same societal expectation as the possession itself.

Monk, et al. (1997), in writing about diagnosis and illness, state:

> Thus, we make sense of our lives in the context of our social history, shaping stories about the groups we belong to and about how we came to be who, how and where we are. Such stories constitute something of our identity; they are the background context that gives the possibility of coherence to our lives. (p. 34)

Crabtree (1997a; 1997b) has advanced the social construction of disorders as an explanation for both MPD/DID and demonic possession. At the core of this argument is that when a person has the need to display their psychic pain, they will do so in a manner that is consistent with what is socially allowed. In describing how mediums enter into their trance states, Goodman (1988b) gives the following description:

> [W]e might speculate that the following process takes place during the training for mediumship. The special breathing techniques and concentration, together with cultural expectation, make it possible for the medium to enter the religious trance; being trained in visualizing departed spirits then enables the medium temporarily to switch off her own [mental] map, making room for another, alien one, namely, that of the possessing spirit. At the dissolution of the trance, the medium's own map once more takes over. (p. 39)

While it would be understood as less common among those who are not trained to enter into such an ASC, it appears that many of those who understand themselves to be involuntarily possessed undergo a similar (albeit unconscious) process to that of mediums or shamans. McGuire and Kantor (1998), in their study of healing practices in suburban New Jersey, note a lack of significantly noticeable ASC among both healers and those seeking to be healed, which would be consistent with cultural beliefs that de-emphasize trance states.

A promotion of the belief in possession and the subsequent need for exorcism can be a way to literally demonize social changes to which an individual or an institution is opposed. It is possible that the dynamic is not obvious to the person involved in the demonization. Examples would include the rejection of the trappings of a modern, disenchanted world by many within a religious community. This can range from the absurd, for example attributing vegetarianism to possession (Hammond & Hammond, 1973; Kiely & McKenna, 2007) to the more serious, as when an exorcist connects the sexual orientation of a stranger to their being possessed (Helmouth, 2014).

CHAPTER SEVEN

BRAIN SCIENCE

Wilkinson (2007) defines the dissociating brain as one which is basically not talking to itself. The conscious brain is now aware of thoughts and behaviors that it does not attribute to itself. This is then interpreted through the client's individual and societal schemas (Kiev, 1969). The cause of this disassociate split may be sexual trauma or other repressed thoughts or experiences (Beyerstein, 1995). This is one explanation for a universal understanding of possession stories.

Wilkinson (2007) further explains some of the symptoms of possession as resulting from bodily reactions: superhuman strength is the result of spikes of adrenaline, speaking foreign language as glossolalia, that is nonsense syllables that mimic language and which itself can be trance-inducing (see Pattison & Casey, 1969), and aversion to religious symbols as acting out of the possession schema. For Beyerstein (1995), the tendency to attribute odd states of consciousness to outside forces is a natural response to a brain which is having difficulty in forming a coherent schema. This phenomenon explains not only spirit possession but also delusional thinking for a number of psychiatric illnesses. Solomon, in quoting a friend, Maggie Robinson, identifies an advantage of mental illness that includes delusions: "You can exorcise the demons of schizophrenics who perceive that there's something foreign inside them. But it's much harder with depressed people because we believe we are seeing the truth. But the truth lies" (2001, p. 129).

Loftus and Ketchum (1994) note that the limbic system of the brain can "misfire", causing hallucinations and emotional responses that can range from the mystical to the terrible, which is a phenomenon that up to 25% of people experience. These experiences are usually understood to be true and meaningful by the people experiencing them. Some go on to productive heights, like medieval mystic and author Hildegard of Bingen (Sachs, 1999) and the science fiction author Philip K. Dick (2011). However, active clinicians regularly treat those whose limbic misfirings do not lead to the heights of creative imaginations but rather significant impairment in living life (Dziegilewski, 2010). Spiegel, et al. (2011) have theorized that people in possession states, like the voluntary trance states of people "speaking in tongues" and hypnotized individuals (both of which have had brain imaging work), may be experiencing an increase in connection within the prefrontal cortex. This would be consistent with brain scans done on individuals who are experiencing DID (Sar, Unal, & Kiziltan, 2001).

Goodman (1988b) was part of a study of the physical effects of ASC by having volunteers listen to drumming for 15 minutes while they assumed positions common in shamanistic rituals. The participants had blood work done. They all had elevated levels of adrenalin, noradrenalin, and cortisol from when they began their involvement in the study, but then their levels dropped. They also had higher levels of beta-endorphin in their blood, which continued after the study was finished. Beta-endorphin is a pain-reducing chemical, which could explain why euphoria often accompanies trance states. They had racing pulses but low blood pressure. When participants were given an EEG, it was discovered that they had theta brain waves with an absence of alpha waves, which would be consistent with the transition from a sleeping to a waking state (Cantero, et al., 2003). Van der Kolk (2014) notes that approximately 80% of children with ADHD and many (although an uncited number) people with PTSD will show high theta and low alpha waves if given an neurofeedback evaluation.

These results have led Goodman (1998b) to conclude that trance states are part of the make-up of the brain for humans, but entering them usually requires some guidance. In doing early brain scans on people with MPD, it has been discovered that different alters of the same person have different brain imaging, whereas a control group of actors doing different characters did not show different imaging when in different characters (Goodman, 1988b).

In a study by Deeley, et al. (2014), 17 volunteers (who were all chosen due to the fact that they were easily hypnotized) were encouraged under suggestion to act out two separate scenarios: an external machine controlling their movements, as well as a machine internally controlling their movements. For the duration of the experiment, they were connected to an fMRI scan. The scans were then compared to persons who were not enacting the scenarios. The results showed few differences in brain functioning if the persons were enacting the scenario of a machine controlling them either externally or internally; however significant differences in brain functioning were seen when compared to the control group. Specifically, the external/internal scans showed an increase in the connections between the primary motor cortex and areas of the brain related to the self in relationship to others. This very preliminary finding does support the theory that possession states allow an individual increased brain functioning to the pre-frontal cortex (Goodman, 1988b; Sar, Unal,& Kiziltan, 2001; Spiegel, et al., 2011).

Anthony Gottlieb (2012) critiques the emphasis on brain science in much contemporary research. His argument, building upon Gazzingia (2011) and Tallis (2011), is that the technology is too young to give definitive results, and the emphasis on the brain minimizes the complexity of human behavior. Graf (2010) has criticized the emphasis on research on brain chemistry, arguing that consciousness is much broader and more inclusive than what can be demonstrated in a scientific way. Marino (2001), specifically writing in terms of depression, claims that the causes are still open for discussion. While Marino recognizes that biochemical reasons for mental health concerns may be the cause, brain chemistry is not exclusive or even necessarily the direct cause of suffering. He claims "pharmaceutical fundamentalists" parallel religious fundamentalists who would pray every mental illness out (Marino, 2001). Frattaroli (2001), who works as a prescribing psychiatrist, allows for the brain imbalance in mental illness but also advocates for a return to a pastoral sense of mental health care as a type of "soul work".

As of this writing, a theory in vogue for a variety of mental health issues is that of Dialectic Behavioral Therapy. DBT has as its origins a way of treating Borderline Personality Disorder, but is being used in a variety of settings now. The originator of the theory, Marsha Linehan (1993), utilized a technique going back to Hegel (1968) of accepting the dialectic, namely a hypothesis will lead to its antithesis, which when reconciled becomes a synthesis. The synthesis is then the new hypothesis. I would like to suggest that what Frattaroli (2001) is doing is such a synthesis; namely admitting that brain based disorders fit for some mental illness, and other people are suffering largely due to other causes, be they social, economic, current or past trauma, or other myriad reasons. A practitioner can jump between these two explanations because the old brain/body divide is purely a construct which is full of obvious holes. This is why good prescribers refer patients who are getting psychiatric medication for some form of therapy.

CHAPTER EIGHT

ADDICTION AND POSSESSION

As mentioned earlier, Rohr (2007) has noted the similarity between addictions and possession. The metaphor of addiction as demonic possession is made directly by the historian Berridge in *Demons: Our Changing Attitudes to Alcohol, Drugs and Tobacco* (2013). Although the book examines an evolving approach from a cultural viewpoint across the US, UK, and Europe, the title exposes the metaphor that many turn to in thinking about substance dependence. As Zoja (1989) argues, the drug addicted youth is a sacrifice that the culture makes to meaninglessness, in the form of unending consumption. It seems fitting that the same rampant consumption that is destroying our world is acted out upon the body of the consumer/addict/possessed sufferer. As such, s/he becomes much like Gerard's (1979, 1989) scapegoat, a concept also utilized in family therapy, especially when examining the family of the addict (see, for example, Satir, 1964). If Zoja (1989) is correct, there might be more than coincidence in the criminal charges that addicts face for drug "possession".

For some from an evangelical or fundamentalist viewpoint, seeing addiction as a form of demonic oppression or possession makes sense. Pat Robertson (b. 1930), perhaps one of the most known Charismatic televangelists and onetime presidential candidate, connected possession with addiction and mental health concerns such as depression (2003). Johnson, a Baptist pastor (2010), advocates avoiding traditional twelve step meetings, in part because they are not religious enough. This approach, which has as part of the focus an emphasis on doctrinal purity, includes the traditional association which is often linked with twelve steps, that addiction is a spiritual disease. It should be noted that Johnson is also a licensed AODA provider. If a person with a substance use disorder is unable to control their use on their own or through the help of their faith community, clinical help is recommended.

Kirby (2006) argues that contemporary media usage leads into a trance state, where a person becomes addicted to the electronic game or the internet. This is certainly a dynamic I see in the field of mental health care currently, especially among a younger set of clients. Numerous participants have made the metaphoric connection of the addicted electronic trance to possession in my group therapy that is a part of our partial hospitalization program.

For overtly post-modern therapists like Harland (1999), the use of metaphor to describe "possession" and "addiction" as well as "dependency" appears almost instinctive. The use is also broad; in this example the author explores: "alcohol, anger, approval, caffeine, chocolate, cleaning, control, diets, drugs, food, gambling, helping, indebtedness, internet, power, relationship, religion, romance, self-harming, sex, shopping, smoking, sugar, television, therapy, etc." (Harland, 1999). Some post-modern theories like Narrative Theory (Eron & Lund, 1996; Monk, et al., 1997; Parry & Doan, 1994) actively encourage patients to re-imagine their experiences in order to gain an increase in their own control, a process that seems the opposite of possession. These approaches also encourage a return to indigenous understandings of illness, if that is what culture (or sub-culture) the patient identifies with. As such, they prefigure the later changes to the DSM-5 (APA, 2013). Other therapists, such as one of my supervisors, understand the addiction as existing like a "demonic presence in the room" which was actively working to undermine the work for the change that both the patient and therapist are seeking to achieve.

Wiseman (2016) claims that crystal methamphetamine is literally a tool of the devil and makes some rather unsubstantiated claims about meth use and Wiccans. For Jung, possession could be seen as a metaphor of the dance of transference and counter-transference:

> The analytic relationship begins to take on the quality of 'possession', being caught 'in the tentacles of an octopus…demonic forces lurking in the darkness. The resultant paradoxical blend of positive and negative, of trust and fear, of hope and doubt, of attraction and repulsion' is the fertile ground, the analytical third from which a new alignment in the personality is effected…the elusive, deceptive, ever-changing content that possesses the patient like a demon now flits about from patient to doctor and, as the third party in the alliance, continues its game, sometime impish and teasing, sometimes really diabolical. (Shenk, 2001, p. 82, quoting Jung, 1966, pp. 179-180, 188)

Jung is further quoted as saying that Hitler was possessed by the collective archetype of the Aryan unconscious (Cumo, 2015b). This extension of the demonic metaphor goes well beyond addictions as demonic and includes the therapy itself, whatever the formal diagnosis.

Messing (1967) documents how Zar practice parallels group therapy for AODA issues, and how alcoholism may be one reason a person becomes involved in the Zar rituals. Often Zar is ritually addressed in a group where everyone has dealt with the possessing spirit, although with various degrees of success. The leader of the group is a person whose recovery is most complete, similar to a mentor or sponsor as well as a leader in an AA group (Alcoholics Anonymous, 1981). Messing (1967) further notes that Zar is a long-term, perhaps even lifelong practice. This has a parallel in many (although not all) models of substance recovery such as Twelve Steps (Stevens & Smith, 2009). Messing (1967) was unclear about long-term recovery and relapse rates and I was unable to find any other evidence about that subject, which in fairness is a similar dynamic in the substance use world. The current approach is to look at recovery as a long-term process similar to other chronic diseases such as asthma and diabetes (National Institute on Drug Abuse, 2014).

Substance use never occurs in a personal or social vacuum; it is always occurring within a context and for a reason. Kiev (1972) notes that substance use may be a "withdrawal from daily stress, for meaningful religious experiences, for psychotherapeutic purposes or for improved functioning in the presence of starvation or oppression" (p. 29). Clinicians who are working cross-culturally, especially in regards to substance use disorders, should take care to be sensitive to both the cultural contexts and the understanding of the substances as well as the personal experiences of the patient in question (SAMSHA, 2014; Straussner, 2001).

Individuals may connect addiction and possession through the therapy process. For some, like the occultist Aleister Crowley, who died as a result of his heroin addiction, it is very overt (Guiley, 2009). But there is a recurrent dynamic among patients who are dealing with addiction that has a spiritual aspect.

SECTION 3

CHAPTER NINE

CONVERSATIONS WITH EXORCISTS

In January 2015, I took some time to interview persons who had experience with possession and exorcisms/deliverance ministries. The three descriptions that follow with Jenny Heckman, "Fr. Tom" and Pastor Brown are from that time. Two years later I saw the documentary *Hostage to the Devil* (Stalker & Marro, 2016) about Malachi Martin. Included in the film is an interview with Laurene Gomez, LMFT, who I reached out to. Our interview is included at the end of this chapter.

Jenny Heckman

I became aware of Jenny when I saw that she had presented to the Wisconsin Counseling Association. The topic of her presentation, working with persons with rigid faith beliefs, grew out of her observation that "conservative faith systems can create an environment that is not conducive to mental health" (Heckman, 2015). Jenny is not antireligious, in fact she is an ordained pastor who reports that she has "worked within the walls of the church since I was 19" (Heckman, 2015). At present she works in her own private practice in Milwaukee, WI as a Licensed Professional Counselor with a very holistic, pastoral perspective.

Jenny identified one specific client who might meet the criteria for possession, who we can call Eve. At present Eve has a Borderline Personality Disorder diagnosis and has previously stated to her mental health providers that she believed herself to be possessed, after which she was placed on antipsychotics. However, Jenny stated that in regard to Eve's claim, "I am not experiencing this as highly delusional" (Heckman, 2015) and it would appear this belief is consistent with Eve's worldview. Jenny reports that she might refer Eve to a pastor for deliverance and/or exorcism, and if Eve requested she would accompany her, although she would not preside at the service. Jenny also felt it would be essential, if this was the situation, to debrief with the client after the ritual was completed. Jenny cited the American Counseling Association's newest Code of Ethics (2014) by saying, "the ACA has made it clear that we are invited, and it is good practice, to learn the language of the person's belief system" (Heckman, 2015).

I asked Jenny if this would be an uncomfortable situation for her to be in or to document, and she stated that previously, "I have had clients ask me to pray over them and anoint them with oil" (Heckman, 2015) as well as having attended outside events that were meaningful for the patient and positive in their therapy, so that her attendance at an exorcism would seem to be a combination of the two. Jenny quickly followed up by stating that in the process her therapeutic goal would be to "have the client see themselves as a whole person and not as divided parts" (Heckman, 2015). She further shared that "we do harm [to our clients] when we feed into the separation" (Heckman, 2015). This therapeutic goal of integration appears to be the same as Jongsma and Peterson's (2006) recommendation in working with patients suffering with DID, and seems a key part of Heckman's orientation.

Jenny Heckman struck me as a very thoughtful and insightful therapist, and her attempt to bridge the world of faith communities (especially evangelical and fundamentalist) and professional mental health practice is just what this book is attempting to do. Among the interviews engaged with exorcists over January, she was the one I most felt on the same page with, although all were very gracious and interesting people.

"Father Tom"

The next interview was with a Catholic priest who asked me not to include his real name. I can say that he is the official exorcist in a Roman Catholic diocese in the Midwest. He has held that particular position since 2000, and he reported that he has yet to perform a full-scale exorcism, although he has seen about 4-5 people a year for deliverance ministry. All of these people have been referred through their existing work with parish priests, so Fr. Tom reports he has had fewer concerns with differential diagnosis as far as mental illness is concerned. When I raised the question of whether such pastoral care could be iatrogenic, he admitted the possibility and cites an early case when he felt the individual was more concerned with attention and may have been "faking her symptoms for the sympathy she would not otherwise get in her life" (Father Tom, 2015). However, Fr. Tom did feel that most of the time, prayer and anointing with oil are a healing and positive experience for a person and he stated "there is no harm in praying over a person" (Fr. Tom, 2015), and it is worth noting that among Catholics and other Christians these actions are increasingly being provided for a multiple of ailments due in part to the influence of the Charismatic movement (see chapter 3 for more on the movement), although not necessarily by an exorcist or even a priest. This type of work seems informed by such Catholic Charismatic writers as Francis MacNutt (Foster, 2008); in fact Fr. Tom and MacNutt both attribute the Catholic Church's struggles with sexual abuse to the social acceptance of homosexuality and MacNutt's wife, Dr. Judith MacNutt, a psychologist, practices a form of religious conversion therapy, even though that has been discredited by the American Psychological Association.

Fr. Tom lives a somewhat reclusive life, as he is officially a hermit, which is consistent with the specific religious order to which he belongs. He was quick to point to some of the older literature on exorcisms, namely Martin (1976), although he also mentioned Fr. Amarth's work (1999). It seemed as if Fr. Tom was intentionally removed from much of the modern world, including his continued use of the prayers of Pope Leo XIII, sometimes in Latin, as opposed to the modern exorcism rite (see Wilkinson, 2007) when he practices his deliverance ministry, although that is a position well within the bounds of formal Catholic practice (Phillips, 2015b). He shared that he is not familiar with more contemporary writings on the subject, which as a hermit is understandable.

Fr. Tom described a theologically conservative viewpoint that described itself as being on the defensive, pointing to the existence of a nearby small-town Masonic Temple as evidence of demonic activity in the area. He also shared stories about the building he lives in having mysterious footprints deep in the floor which he attributes to the devil and not a careless builder. Fr. Tom stated that once he was visited by a Protestant police officer who claimed that Fr. Tom's ministry was helping to scare away Satanic Ritual Abuse (SRA) in the area, although there has never been any substantiated reports of such activity (see, for example, Cuneo, 2001 on SRA). Fr. Tom also reported that he buys "Little Devil" brand skateboards when he is in stores (which, as a hermit, is not all that often) because they had a contract to sell the buyer's soul to the devil in exchange for "time away from homework". In doing so he felt that he was keeping kids away from that temptation; however, it would also appear he is (in a small way) feeding into the marketing scheme of the company.

It should be emphasized that Fr. Tom tended to focus his energy not on the dark or Satanic, and he shared that "all exorcists agree, confession is more powerful than an exorcism" (Fr. Tom, 2015). In addition to being a hermit and an exorcist, he is a chaplain to an order of nuns, does spiritual direction for an area seminary, and has other duties with the diocese. This is not to say that he did not see the very real presence of evil in the world; however, he did share that he keeps a watchful eye for when people attribute every ill and misfortune to demonic origins.

While I was leaving this interview, Fr. Tom gathered some information for me in a folder. It included a chapter by Martin (1976), some newsletters of ministries he is involved in (all very non-descript), and two photocopied sheets without authors. The titles of the sheets were "Ruler Demons" and "Repressed Spirits", and both consisted of long lists of nouns and verbs. These included some obvious aspects one would expect from an exorcist, like witchcraft, pride, occult activity; as well as some very clearly mental health related aspects such as schizophrenia, delusions of grandeur, and paranoia.

Fr. Tom also claimed to have some skills analyzing handwriting. He examined my notes and described a person who bore very little resemblance to me. All in all, I did find him to be a very pastoral and gentle soul, but we clearly had a very different take on the world.

Perry Brown

Pastor Jenny Heckman had given me information about Pastor Perry Brown, who I was easily able to connect with. He is by training a carpenter who felt a greater call to serve and ended up on the board of directors of Hope Ministry, which at the time was a transitional housing program in Milwaukee, WI for people "ravaged by addiction" (Brown, 2015). After a number of years, Pastor Perry accepted the directorship of the ministry and rebranded it from a traditional transitional housing program to what is now known as a "greenhouse for people" (Brown, 2015). As part of that transition, the ministry focused on one location, a former hotel which can house around 40 people, as well as broadening their participation from people struggling with strict AODA issues to include other issues, such as process addictions and trauma histories. Pastor Perry did state that the vast majority still are people who are "broken from their addictions" (Brown, 2015) but that a focus of their work has been a holistic approach to help people "live, learn and develop new habits" (Brown, 2015). As part of the transition from traditional transitional housing to being a "greenhouse for people" they have encouraged families to reunite and move in.

The reason Jenny Heckman had suggested I contact Pastor Brown was in relation to one of these reunited families. A father, who had been a resident of Hope Ministry for a while, was able to get custody of his 12-year-old daughter, who we will call Faith. The girl had become involved with Child Protective Services due to her mother's inability to effectively parent due to her addictions. During the time when the mother had custody, "Faith" was sexually abused by her mother as well as other men, and she may have been prostituted in order for mom to score drugs. Soon after moving in with her father at Hope Ministry, Faith's significant mental health issues became apparent. One day she was tearing apart her apartment that she shared with her dad. Police were called to restrain her.

Faith was subsequently hospitalized and given diagnoses of Post-Traumatic Stress Disorder (PTSD) as well as Oppositional Defiant Disorder (ODD). During the hospitalization, Pastor Perry reports he had a vision of her face in a tile floor and felt a spiritual presence which he thought seemed demonic. He visited her in the hospital and, he said without prompting, she told him "Pastor, I have a demon" (Brown, 2015). Pastor Brown said a prayer of deliverance over her in the hospital and that afterword, both felt a sense of calm. Since then, Brown reports Faith has had experiences with others you would expect from a 12-year-old with a difficult background, but nothing near the level of what initiated her hospitalization.

Perry Brown shared another deliverance that he had performed, also with a young person. This person, "Chris", had apparently been reading a book about how looking at clouds can help when calling up spirits. Ironically, when Pastor Brown met Chris it felt to Perry like "blocks of concrete were on my shoulders" (Brown, 2015), a feeling that stayed through the night. He reports that upon giving a deliverance prayer, the feeling departed. It is interesting to note the similarity between Pastor Brown's description of Chris opening himself to demonic powers through the cloud book (which he did not specifically name) and M. Scott Peck's (2005) description of both Jersey's and Becca's youthful readings as opening them up to the power of the devil.

Pastor Brown had tremendous energy and spoke with clear passion and intelligence, but also without any apparent formal training in theology or in pastoral ministry. Such a position could result in negative consequences for an exorcism gone wrong. However, in his description of his actual deliverance prayers, no acts of coercion were engaged in. He described only direct spontaneous prayer and then only after asking and being given permission from the other person. This is the same sort of action I could imagine him doing for any illness, any sin, or even a personal loss. Within his personal theology, informed by a close reading of the Bible, it seems all these fit within the continuum of human experience. It was clear that he takes his vocation seriously, and like the other two interviews, clearly felt a sense of caring and importance in the ministry that he is active in.

In reflecting upon the interviews with the three exorcists, all recognized an existence of evil in the world which could manifest in very personal ways. This differs from a more typically liberal theological orientation, which tends to identify evil as more structural (i.e. the sins of racism and structural inequality). This seems to explain why there are very few

Christian exorcisms from what are known as mainline denominations. For conservative Christians, a tension exists between the perceived omnipotence of the Divine and the perceived power of the demonic, including over the baptized. Pastor Heckman addressed this tension by stating, "I believe that if someone is sealed in Christ, the powers of darkness cannot completely take control, however people who perpetuate repeated trauma are dehumanizing another, and that feels different, it seems an element of something dark" (Heckman, 2015). For Heckman, there is a melding of structural evil (in the sense of patterns of repeated trauma) with personal sin. In this, she shows a more liberal theological understanding than either Pastor Brown or Fr. Tom, which is an assessment I believe all three would agree with. This is not to claim that all conservative theological orientations or persons dismiss the existence of structural evil, but rather to suggest that liberal theologies minimize or dismiss personal evil. A consistent point raised by all three was that this is a dangerous worldview. Personally, I find it uncomfortable to claim a belief in Satan. However, it is hard to dismiss Heckman's (2015) example of repeated trauma upon a person as something other than evil. Furthermore, the reported benefits of each moment of deliverance, although impossible to follow up and verify, do appear to have caused no harm to the person involved and may have helped in some way.

Laurene Gomez, LMFT

Laurene was featured in the documentary *Hostage to the Devil* (Stalker & Marro, 2016) which focused primarily on Malachi Martin (see pp. 107-108 of this book); although she admitted she had only met the man once and found him "fascinating" (Gomez, 2017). She became interested in this work through her own personal spiritual journey, growing up Roman Catholic but deeply questioning some aspects of the church's practice, such as "why are people sad at funerals" (Gomez, 2017). This led her to extensive reading into spiritual matters and world religions; she joked that while other people were out having fun on a Friday night she would be buried in the library (which I must admit is also my idea of a good night). While she was finishing up her master's degree in marriage and family therapy (which, like all mental health professions, requires a lengthy practicum and internship), she became connected to Ed and Lorraine Warren (see pages 105-106 of this book). One of her roles was to provide a mental health perspective on the reports of those who were suffering. Laurene states that she worked to differentiate those whose experiences were clearly grounded in mental health as well as to continue to work with the family after they went through any rituals, in order to have a longer term and holistic approach to their healing (Gomez, 2017). As the work of the Warrens became more widely known, she would be invited to participate in many exorcisms, including by traditional Catholics. She stated that she had been involved in "more exorcisms than I can count, into the hundreds" (Gomez, 2017).

I asked Laurene to describe some of her experiences in her role, given there does seem to be such a difference between the mundane (albeit therapeutic) work Fr. Tom described above and which Cuneo (2001) observed, and the lurid descriptions that occur not only in Hollywood but also in the more widely read works of those like Martin (1976). She did state she had never seen levitation or vomiting of pea soup but she did have times when the room would become very cold, "a chill that would stay with you long after the exorcism was over. This was usually around when, during the Rite, the demon is asked what its name is" (Gomez, 2017). Laurene also stated that she would experience the three classic signs of demonic possession, including knowledge of things otherwise unknown (including such things as occurrences in her morning or information about her colleagues), superhuman strength in ways she states could not just be explained by simple adrenaline surges (justifying restraints to protect both the possessed and the exorcism team), and a change in language. She did state that it was not necessarily speaking in a foreign tongue by the possessed person but rather, the demon would speak in a guttural voice and there would be simultaneously other voices speaking at the same time (Gomez, 2017).

Laurene, who now divides her professional work between a state hospital, including a forensic wing which works with those who are "not guilt for reasons of insanity" and private practice, has seen a change in the way mental health providers are more open to a variety of modalities in people's recovery. "When I started 20 years ago, no one would have been able to recommend yoga, hypnosis, or supplements, which now is fairly standard" (Gomez, 2017). She was clear that recognition of the dark side of spirituality, including demonic possession, is not readily accepted among her peers. However, she felt more comfortable being interviewed in documentaries (and for this book) in part because she knew she was coming close to retirement. "It is a liberating feeling", she shared with a laugh (Gomez, 2017). Laurene felt her work is based in helping people embrace their true selves:

> I try and help people rediscover who they really are, and that is when the other pieces, such as their marriage or childrearing, tend to click into place. If they love exercising, I encourage them to return to exercising. If they had a rich prayer life, whatever they called who they prayed to, God, Allah,

> nature, I worked with them to reconnect with what gave them strength. It is when we lose connection that we become open to these negative things and we suffer. (Gomez, 2017, n.p.)

Laurene, much like Jenny Heckman, was a warm and interesting person who had a very broad and accepting take on others and their path to recovery, in whatever way that seemed to show up. I should state that my sympathy and ease with talking with both of them over the phone should also be balanced by all three of us being in similar mental health fields, something I just did not share with Pastor Brown or Fr. Tom, although they were also warm and gracious and very grounded.

CHAPTER TEN

CONTEMPORARY TREATMENT

Among mental health professionals, Burke (2011) identifies three opinions about possession states and exorcisms:

1. they are inherently false and harmful,
2. they exist as a placebo, or
3. they are real and may have therapeutic value.

Following the first line of argument is a case study from Madrid, Spain where a patient with schizophrenia discontinued medication in favor of multiple exorcisms by Catholic priests, reportedly disrupting the traditional mental health treatment (Tajima-Pozo, et al., 2005). Neki, et al. (1986) state that a referral to a folk healer or exorcist is never justified but encourage mental health professionals to discuss the similarities and the differences in the approaches with the patient. Hardtke (2015) raises the ethical dilemma of how deaths that have occurred during exorcisms should give pause to those who believe in the efficacy of exorcisms.

Building from the first argument, that exorcisms are essentially harmful to clients, several mental health professionals have had difficulty due to their involvement in exorcisms. One, Kenneth Olson, a psychologist in Arizona, had rather surprisingly billed the state's Child Protective Services for providing the service. Several others have had their professional licenses revoked, including in Missouri and Tennessee, for being involved in some form with exorcisms with their clients (Thomason, 2008).

However, in an approach that blends the second and third lines of argument, Field (1955) was one of the first to seriously examine the positive approaches of traditional rituals in patients suffering from psychological issues. Kiev (1973) advocates for clients from cultures which believe in spirit possession to participate in rituals that purge evil spirits, drawing parallels with the social support of groups like Alcoholics Anonymous. One unique advantage to such cultic activities is the integration of an ecstatic emotional and spiritual element which is all too often missing from Western mental health approaches (see also Good, 1994; Kleinman, 1981). Fox

(1967) writes about the healing ceremonies of indigenous communities in rural Philippines who, in the midst of illness, challenge their possessing demon to perform a song and dance through the work of a shaman, and then will repeat the routine in social gatherings from that point on.

When thinking about culturally competent treatment, it should be noted that it is the client who determines what is culturally competent, and not the provider (SAMSHA, 2007). It is also worth noting that such concepts as a cultural-bound syndrome may be more an intellectual construct among professionals than a "real-world" experience; when Ross, Schroeder, and Ness (2013) surveyed patients in a psychiatric hospital in the US, they found a large number of the Caucasian patients manifesting the symptoms but not the formal diagnoses of worldwide "cultural-bound syndromes" like possession, *amok* (a condition which has entered into common parlance as "running amok)" and *latah,* that is dissociation after a sudden fright, included in the DSM-IV TR (APA, 1994) but not included in the DSM-5 (APA, 2013).

Aho (2008) advocates understanding a client's experiences from the client's own worldview. Their symptoms may make sense in their own perspective, so treatment can integrate these understandings, as was the case when Pattison (1971) created the space for the family to exorcise the demon possessing Mary. Somasundaram, Thivakaran, and Bhugra (2008) compared the treatment approaches of three distinct groups in Northern Sri Lanka. Group A consisted of 30 psychiatric residents who complained of having a possession state which was unwanted and sought Western modalities. Group B consisted of 30 people who identified being possessed and pursued their treatment through religious practice. Group C was composed of 30 people who went to the hospital for other issues having no complaints related to possession (control). It was found that those who pursued a traditional approach fared as well as those who pursued a Western approach, indicating that, within this small sample at least, folk exorcism can be as effective as psychiatric hospitalization. It would be very interesting if such a study were to be repeated in the US or another Western country, given the significant cultural differences between the US and Sri Lanka.

Field (1955) documents cases of "in-patient" treatment in the African Gold Coast. The patients all believed they were possessed and/or bewitched. In one case, the woman who was supposedly bewitched as well as the victim were treated together; eventually the "witch" blessed the victim, who quickly then recovered. Laubscher (1937) documents how, among the Tembu people of South Africa, bewitched people attempt to join the people who live "under the water" after hearing them call to them. If they are saved by their tribe from drowning, they are kept with "witch doctors" known as *ukutwasa* for up to several years, possibly becoming *ukutwasa* themselves. Recovery rates are said to be high, and at the time of writing that text, the patients were hidden from European colonial authorities, for fear they would be treated in a Western manner, which was seen as much less successful. Lambo (1957), a Nigerian practitioner who was trained in Western psychology, advocated that when working with the Yoruba people, cases of possession and bewitchment should be treated traditionally.

Van Duijl, Kleijn, and de Jong (2014) studied 119 people who believed they were suffering a possessed state in southwestern Uganda. They found 1/3 had a decrease in symptoms with Western approaches (i.e. medicine and talk therapy), whereas 99% had a significant decrease in symptoms during the study when going to traditional healers for a culturally sanctioned exorcism, a truly remarkable and profound difference in recovery rates, although one which does not seem to be repeated in such drastic results among other studies. In a recent case among mountain climbers, Khan and Sahni (2013) report on an exorcism of a 20-year-old female who began to channel the spirit of a former deceased climber. The authors report the exorcism was successful and at that time of writing, the patient had not experienced any other mental health symptoms before or after the climb.

Watters (2011) has shown that, if culturally sanctioned, exorcisms can have higher rates of healing for clients than Western approaches, at least for schizophrenia. Dein and Samad Illaiee (2009) do suggest that clinicians check to see if such beliefs as reported by clients are consistent with cultural worldviews, otherwise some examples of psychosis could be missed.

Sometimes the notion of a solid and definable worldview is itself a challenge. Contemporary memoirs abound in describing those who are searching for a larger perspective, and often include some form of hybrid or idiosyncratic approach. Faith Salie (2016), a frequent National Public Radio personality, recently wrote about her divorce after her husband, among other complaints, felt she was possessed by Satan. In the chapter entitled "The Exorcism", she humorously recounts a yoga-based retreat led by several African American women where she was able, through washing off her mud-covered body in extremely hot water, to "exorcise" not the devil but her undealt-with grief over the loss of her mother. She writes, "I didn't quite know it at the time, but I had been reborn. [My husband] didn't quite know it, but he'd exorcised me out of his life. And though it would take a while, I was starting to possess myself" (p. 85)

Irmak (2014), a Turkish mental health practitioner, not only sees the value in exorcisms as part of folk healing for schizophrenia, he also agrees with the traditional etiology which attributes classic symptoms such as hallucinations as a misinterpretation of demonic forces. This position generated some negative responses in a blog dedicated to maintaining the materialistic basis of scientific inquiry (Karlsson, 2015a). I contacted Karlsson and asked, if we remove Irmak's (2014) attribution of schizophrenia to demonic forces and instead looked at Watters' findings of cultural efficacy in treating schizophrenia as possession (2011), would the same critique be valid? In response, Karlsson (2015b) replied that the "perceived benefit of traditional cultural treatments has to be demonstrated to be better than placebo (both in terms of the treatment effect and the cultural benefit), the risks have to be adequately assessed and compared with the benefits and the effects of combining science-based and superstition-based treatments have to be understood… If the cultural traditions had a clear medical benefit, it would be just called 'medicine' and not 'cultural traditions'" (n.p.). In the comments section, Karlsson replied with a parallel, "would a person who was bitten by a snake be seen by a shaman or a doctor?" (2015b, n.p.). The gap in this line of reasoning is that the snake bite is an acute situation, whereas schizophrenia is a chronic lifelong condition that affects how a person interacts with their society. If we move beyond a doctor/shaman dichotomy and encourage the best medicine as well as the best integrative approaches (some form of talk therapy/traditional healing/case management), the patient with schizophrenia seems to have a better chance by pursuing a both/and approach. The patient with a snake bite does not have a chance if the poison or infections are not addressed medically; although later cultural healing may be helpful or essential if such a bite had a cultural implication, such as ritual impurity. Such a blending appears in Newberg (2012), who tells about a patient who saw a doctor for malaria and then a shaman to address why she had the bad luck of being bitten by the infected insect. This overcoming of the dichotomy appears to be done by the writings of Lewis Mehl-Madrona (e.g. 2003, 2008), who is a medical doctor and psychiatrist as well as a tribal shaman from Cree, Cherokee, and Lakota backgrounds. His medical work includes obvious Western allopathic (i.e. standard) approaches as well as working with patients to develop rituals that are meaningful for them, and giving them the time to share in visits with their doctor.

Crabtree (1997a) claims as a therapist to have worked with about 50 people who have experiences of possession. He does not venture into determining the objective truth of the possession, but rather focuses on the personal experience of the patient, drawing a parallel with hallucinations by a patient. He divides his reportedly possessed patients into 4 different categories: possession by the deceased, usually family members (similar to those reported by McAll, 1981 and McKenna & Kiely, 2007); possession by the living; possession by a "group mind" (such as cults, see also Crabtree 1997b for more, including ideologies and families as a "group mind"); and possession puzzles, which do not fit other categories. Interestingly, Crabtree (1997a; 1997b) does not discuss *demonic* possession among his 50 patients (although he certainly discussed it in other parts of the book looking at the history of possession). Among those with whom he has worked is one person who believed they were possessed by a pagan deity and another person possessed by a sprite. Under the first category, those possessed by a deceased family member were, all but one, females who had previously suffered sexual abuse by men. The other exception was a woman who had a sister very close in age with severe challenges both physically and mentally. It would appear that this phenomenon of possession by the spirit of a family member is more reported in the British Isles and parts of Canada (which is where Crabtree is writing). In the description of the exorcisms, it is completely possible that all of the stories are personally meaningful to the patient in question, but there was no definitive proof of an outside spirit presence. Also worthy of note is the use by Crabtree of hypnosis techniques, which have been shown to have a high level of iatrogenic effects due to the suggestions of the hypnotist.

Baglio (2009) encourages priests to consult with mental health professionals in diagnosing clients, but adds the caveat that only if the clinician believes in the possibility of possession. Goodman (1988b) strongly advocates the therapeutic use of exorcism. Allison and Schwartz (1980) note that in several cases of patients diagnosed with MPD, exorcisms were successful in alleviating some of the symptoms. It is interesting to note that one of the patients Allison treated had an initial possession incredibly similar to the opening of Martin's (1976) book on possession, a fact which Allison and Schwartz (1980) do not comment upon but which lends some level of suspicion to either the patient's reporting or the writing of the text.

Diamond (2011), a forensic psychologist who writes for the popular magazine *Psychology Today*, has commented on the popularity of possession narratives in films and in society. He makes the connection between psychotherapy and exorcism but stops short of advocating for patients to undergo exorcisms. Instead, he advocates for providers to be able to accommodate those who believe themselves to be possessed, although it is unclear how he would go about that.

For patients with DID, Bull (2001) found that exorcism can be helpful, but only if it fits with the client's worldview and is done in a non-coercive manner. It can be harmful if done with coercion. In a review of treatment done on 15 Christian evangelical and/or fundamentalist patients with a DID diagnosis who had received one or more exorcisms, there were generally positive reactions and outcomes, especially if they found congruence between the style of exorcism and their own belief system (Bull, Ellasan, and Ross, 1998). From a Christian fundamentalist as well as mental health therapist viewpoint, Page (1989) does allow for exorcism as a therapeutic technique, but urges caution from both a clinical and theological viewpoint.

Cuneo (2001) interviewed several practicing mental health professionals who refer clients for exorcisms. All of the mental health workers felt a degree of professional distrust to hostility from their colleagues at the very notion of referring a patient for an exorcism. Cuneo (2001) has noticed that out of the 50 exorcisms he witnessed, some people have experienced a lessening of or an end to their symptoms. He does note that his study did not follow up to determine the length of relief for those who were suffering. He also raised the issue of how the exorcism is approached: is it done coercively, for the wrong reasons, is it a danger to anyone? If yes, then it should not proceed. However, consensual and therapeutic exorcisms appear to have real benefit in his research.

Rosik (2003) questioned 6 religiously sensitive practitioners with expertise in DID about the therapeutic use of exorcism and found a wide variation in responses. All were agreed that faith communities can be supportive of patients, and have not done enough in the past to create a community of healing. But even among those who did believe exorcisms can have a place in treatment, there was a difference in identifying the threshold of symptoms to warrant either an exorcism or a deliverance prayer. In an earlier work Rosik (1997), in both personal experience and research, found evidence wanting for the efficacy of exorcisms and further warns that they may be harmful at times. There is a fear that exorcisms with people who have psychiatric illness can convince the sufferers that their issues are spiritual as opposed to psychological, further complicating or jeopardizing future treatment (see also Baglio, 2009). While writing from a public health perspective in rural Nepal, Sapkota, et al. (2014) found value in looking at possession as potentially meaningful for the patients in explaining a variety of mental health ailments (anxiety, depression, PTSD), but they also warn about iatrogenic consequences. This is paralleled with the phenomenon that Nicholas Spanos (1991) noted, where once a client is encouraged to have multiple personalities; it is difficult to stop that behavior.

Midelfort (2005) has noted the lack of success that mental health practitioners have had with engaging in exorcisms themselves. The extreme manifestation of malfeasance and a patient's untimely death have been reported as occurring during exorcisms, although not while a mental health practitioner was involved, albeit that is until recently, a rarely reported phenomenon (Cuneo, 2001; Goodman, 1988b; Kiely & McKenna, 2007; Wilkinson, 2007).

Midelfort (2005) parses out the significant difference between the understanding of unwanted spirit possession, which requires the same basic exorcism, and a psycho-medical condition, which may be responsive to medication, talk therapy, or a behavioral remedy. Under the medical model, any efficacy of an exorcism would be attributed to the placebo effect, which may be a way of dismissing it (Cohen, 2002). Kottler (2003) argues that within medicine itself, the belief in the effectiveness by the patient and the practitioner is often very powerful and cannot be separated from the treatment outcome. Midelfort (2005) points out that the exorcist is usually operating within the same worldview as the possessed, and any healing that is offered through the ritual occurs within a larger social context. This is borne out in Wilkinson's (2007) conversations with Italians who had reported being possessed and exorcised. Several of these individuals reported feeling a sense of relief that they were possessed and not mentally ill. Wilkinson (2007) cites Dr. Mastronardi, an Italian expert on psychopathology, who sees the behavior of priests in exorcisms as, "characterized by humanity and empathy, freely expressed by physical contact, hugs, stroking, affectionate gestures, placing on of hands, etc. (something which is sought after by these patients). This is something a therapist cannot do . . ." (p. 154).

Exorcism may work on the dichotomy between healing and curing, if healing is understood as bringing a person back into the right relationship with the self and their world, while curing is an ending of a disease (Crossan, 1999; Kleinman, 1981). For Lewis (1986/2003), it is the emotionally and spiritually charged nature of exorcism that is an integral part of the change that can occur in a patient, which is in direct contrast to a detached and controlled experience of Western medicine. Baglio (2009) writes that one of the possible benefits of possession and exorcism for clients, when compared to Western approaches, is social expectation (a point reiterated by Wilkinson, 2007). For Dr. Steven Jay Lynn (Baglio, 2009), there is possible damage caused in DID patients in dredging up memories (which may be false) through talk therapy, but an exorcism allows a clean break. Van Duijl, Kleijn, and de Jong (2014), in their study of Ugandans experiencing possession states, note that exorcisms allowed the people to see a decrease in their symptoms (or the disappearance of the possessing spirit entirely) without having to deal with traumatic past issues.

Craig Isaacs (2010), an Anglican priest and a psychiatrist, believes that there are times when a person who appears initially to be mentally ill may in fact be possessed by an outside spirit. He holds to a tripartite nature of the person, body-soul-spirit, that is similar to the Jungian writer James Hillman (1991). For Isaacs (2010), body illness is treated through medicine, soul illness is treated through mental health psychological care, and spiritual illness (including possession) is treated through a religious rite, usually personal repentance for sin or exorcism to rid the person of the demonic presence. Piedmont, Village, and Dien (1987) document in interviews of 30 Bangladeshi immigrants to the UK who had been hospitalized for various psychiatric issues (as well as interviews with each of their case workers) how both Western psychiatric care and traditional exorcisms were mutually helpful in stabilizing their symptoms.

Placebos (Latin for "I shall please") work in a variety of situations, as documented in Jacobs (2012). As Pipher (2003) wrote:

> Traditional healers and customs work because they are believed to work. Almost all mental health cures involve placebo effects. In therapy people improved partly because they expect to improve. They count on what a Vietnamese boy I met at a high school described as, 'The beauty and mystery of hope'. (p. 167)

Debra Murray, PhD (2015), at a training course I attended, recently described placebos as the "installation of hope". Placebos certainly seem more effective when the patient believes in what is happening, but there is evidence that there is some degree of effectiveness even if the patient does not believe in the treatment (Jacobs, 2012). Baglio (2009) reports on Michael Hyland, a psychologist who studies placebos (or, as he calls them, therapeutic rituals). Hyland began to study them in order to understand why psychotherapy works. He argues that placebos have a dual function, one is the widely understood response expectancy ("I expect the treatment to work, therefore it does"). The other function is that the person is a dynamic being whose needs begin to be met in the process of the healing encounter. This reinforces their involvement in the process, helping the person, in Hyland's terms, "with self-defining or self-actualizing goals" (Baglio, 2009, p. 203).

McGuire, a sociologist, studied healing rituals in suburban Essex County, New Jersey in the early 1980s (McGuire & Kantor, 1998). In this qualitative study, 313 respondents were asked about the use of allopathic (i.e. Mainstream Western medicine) and other forms of healing, including prayer groups. These responses were compared to a smaller control group. Among participants in Charismatic healing prayer groups, there was concern expressed about those who pursued healing from non-Christian healers (for this group, this included the Christian Scientist denomination), as that opened up a person to the need for deliverance or exorcism.

A clinician ought to examine if the supernatural explanations are an attempt to avoid assigned blame. Some psychological problems can be attributed to curses by people who believe in exorcisms, especially in places like Italy. Fr. Amorth, the famous Vatican exorcist, was said to have been disappointed that the post-Vatican II changes to the Catholic exorcism rite explicitly forbid its use in instances when a curse is believed to be the cause of the possession (Guiley, 2009). Issues like depression, physical illness, divorce, financial woes, and suicide have been blamed on spiritual forces, as opposed to other natural explanations (Baglio, 2009). Hale (2009) notes an ancient emphasis going back to the days of the Roman Empire and the use of 'curse tablets' to bewitch horses at the racetrack, a tradition which continues with worries of modern-day curses.

CHAPTER ELEVEN

CONCLUSION

Many people, from a variety of cultures, believe in unwanted possession. The most recent change to the DSM-5 (APA, 2013) now allows for a client who believes they are possessed by an outside spirit to be classified as having Dissociative Identity Disorder, DID. This change brings the DSM more in line with the International Classification of Disease (ICD) diagnosis F44.89 "Other Dissociative and Conversion Disorders, due to trance or possession state" (www.icd10data.com, 2013). While many contemporary Western providers may not believe such a condition to be caused by outside non-human entities, During, et al. (2011) predict an increase in the reports of possession, due in part to immigration, although as has been shown, changes in current spiritual worldviews will play a part as well. Burke (2011) and Cuneo (2001) already note an increase in reports of possession and in subsequent exorcisms, not only among immigrant communities but also among Westerners of various faith traditions.

Allowing such an understanding of possession as both a personal and cultural schema for disease is a change that further allows clinicians to treat persons who believe they are possessed in a culturally competent manner, collaborating with religious/cultural figures in the client's life, or referring a client to a person who may perform an exorcism, presuming such a performance is safe for the client and is not believed to make their suffering worse. Such referrals or collaboration should only be made

1. if the client believes themselves to be possessed and in need of an exorcism without coercion from the therapist or others,
2. they have a belief system that is consistent with belief in possession states (versus clear forms of psychosis) and most importantly,
3. the ritual is performed in a safe and respectful manner, causing no harm to the person involved.

Looking at the results of Peck's (1998, 2005) in-office exorcisms and the findings of other therapists who engaged in exorcisms for therapeutic purposes (Midelfort, 2005; Rosik, 1997; 2003), it does not appear to be beneficial for a therapist to personally engage in the rite. Personally, when I reflect upon those who I thought might benefit from a discussion of possession, even metaphorically, I did not recommend or mention it because that is not how the patient understood their suffering. Moving forward in my clinical practice, that hesitation will undoubtedly continue.

Given the recommendations for Roman Catholic exorcists to collaborate with mental health providers (Baglio, 2005; Wilkinson, 2007) as well as the problems that have occurred in other denominations, and the increasing acceptance of some aspects of mental healthcare among "traditional" communities that had previously felt resistance to contemporary mental health approaches (Cuneo, 2001), it is possible that a clinician would be in a situation where such a referral could be made to them from a member of the clergy. Previously, such a recommendation was felt by some to be somehow outside the pale of acceptable practice, and therapists would not announce such activities to their colleagues even if they did engage in such collaborations, as cited in the conclusion of Cuneo's book (2001) and in the interview with Gomez (2017). Now, individual therapists will be forced in such a situation to decide if a referral for an exorcism is beneficial for the individual, or if the rite might cause further harm, either through ignoring non-spiritual explanations for the symptoms or feeding into existing pathologies and delusions. Hopefully, the change in the DSM-5 (APA, 2013) will open up the office conversation to include such a referral when it is seen as potentially helpful.

Dein and Samad Illaiee (2009) caution that when working cross-culturally, clinicians do not attribute all seemingly bizarre beliefs as culturally based, as true cases of psychosis can in that situation be missed. Personally, I have two clients who seem to be examples of such differences. One is a woman from one of the local indigenous tribes who believes she is being called to be a medicine woman, a role she does not want to play. She has been woken by "the spirits" on multiple occasions, but reports that other members of her family have experienced the same phenomenon. In her case, I continued to see her for the pre-existing depression and anxiety and encouraged her to be active with traditional healings with the native community she had already connected with. In the second case, a woman I was working with had a formal diagnosis of Major Depressive Disorder with psychotic features as well as Borderline Personality Disorder. She had previously had an exorcism performed by a member of the Seventh Day Adventist congregation she was somewhat active with. This was interesting as the denomination has attempted to distance itself from exorcism, and has objected that the church has been unfairly connected to exorcisms that were done by former members of the fold in France (www.news.adventist.org, n.d.). In her case, her exorcism seemed to have caused little harm but also was of little help given that she continued to struggle with her mental health.

The referral to a religious leader is an individual clinical decision which includes the suffering persons' perspective and worldview, but also those of the clinician. Ethically, no clinician can be expected to refer someone for an exorcism if they believe such a referral would be harmful or counterproductive. However, even if the clinician doubts the validity of the exorcism (for example, rejecting the "soul theory"), there may be times when such a referral would be a beneficial practice for therapy. The proposed changes give a greater allowance for a clinician to recommend such a procedure without fear of professional reprisal or scorn. It would appear that this change will bring into the open some mental health care providers who were "closeted" about their referrals for exorcisms.

ACKNOWLEDGEMENTS

This book began as my master's thesis and I found the material too fascinating to put away, so I kept at it over the years. Thanks go to the Journal of Exceptional Experiences and Psychology (https://issuu.com/exceptionalpsychology), which published an early version as an essay and which graciously allowed republication in a greatly expanded form. Of course, the faculty at Winona State University was key to my journey to being a mental health professional, and this work owes a great debt especially to Drs. Roni Johnson, Jo Hittner and Cyndi Briggs. I also wish to thank those who took the time to be interviewed, Jenny Heckman, Perry Brown, Laurene Gomez and "Fr. Tom". Finally, I wish to thank my family, especially my "little devils" Sebastian and Beatrice.

REFERENCES

Aaronovitch, D. (2010). *Voodoo histories: The role of conspiracy theory in shaping modern history*. Riverhead: New York.

Achebe, C. (1959). *Things fall apart*. London: Heinemann.

Adinkrah, M. (2011). "Child witch hunts in contemporary Ghana." *Child Abuse & Neglect, 35* (*9*): 741-752.

Adler, G. [Producer]; Aguilar, M. [Producer]; & Lawrence, F. (2005). *Constantine* [Motion Picture.] USA: Warner Brothers.

Aho, K. (2008). "Medicalizing mental health: A phenomenological alternative." *Journal of Medical Humanities*, *29*, 243-259.

Alberge, D. (2016). "Christopher Marlowe credited as one of Shakespeare's co-writers." *The Guardian*. Retrieved on October 24, 2016 from: https://www.theguardian.com/culture/2016/oct/23/christopher-marlowe-credited-as-one-of-shakespeares-co-writers?utm_source=esp&utm_medium=Email&utm_campaign=GU+Today+USA+-+morning+briefing+2016&utm_term=196262&subid=14329163&CMP=ema_a-morning-briefing_b-morning-briefing_c-US_d-1.

Alcoholics Anonymous. (1981). *Twelve steps and twelve traditions*. New York: Alcoholics Anonymous World Services.

Al-Habeeb, T.A. (2003). "A pilot study of faith healers' views on evil eye, jinn possession, and magic in the kingdom of Saudi Arabia." *Journal of Family & Community Medicine*, *10* (*3*): 31-38.

Alexie, S. (1995). *Reservation blues*. New York: Grove.

Allen, T.B. (1993). *Possessed: The true story of an exorcism*. New York: Doubleday.

Allison, R.B., & Schwartz, T. (1980). *Minds in many pieces*. New York: Rawson, Wade.

Amarth, G. (1999). *An exorcist tells his story*. San Francisco: Ignatius Press.

Ambrose, S.A. (1996). *Crazy Horse and Custer: The parallel lives of two American warriors*. New York: New York.

American Counseling Association. (2014). *ACA code of ethics*. Alexandria, VA: American Counseling Association.

American Psychological Association. (2008). "Answers to your questions for a better understanding of sexual orientation and homosexuality." Retrieved from https://www.apa.org/topics/lgbt/orientation.pdf on January 26, 2016.

American Psychiatric Association. (1980). *The diagnostic and statistical manual of mental disorders*. Third Edition. Arlington, VA: American Psychiatric Association.

—. (1994). *The diagnostic and statistical manual of mental disorders*. Fourth Edition. Arlington, VA: American Psychiatric Association.

—. (2000). *The diagnostic and statistical manual of mental disorders*. Fourth Edition, text revision. Arlington, VA: American Psychiatric Association.

—. (2013). *The diagnostic and statistical manual of mental disorders*. 5th Edition. Arlington, VA: American Psychiatric Association.

Anson, J. (1977). *The Amityville horror: A true story*. New York: Pocket Star.

Aquinas, T. (2003). *On evil*. Trans. R. Regan. Oxford: Oxford University Press.

Aristotle. (1984). *The complete works of Aristotle: The revised Oxford translation*. Ed. J. Barnes. Princeton, NJ: Princeton University Press.

Arkoff, S.Z. (Producer) & Rosenberg, S. [Director]. (1979). *The Amityville horror* [Motion Picture]. USA: American International Pictures.

Armstrong, K. (2002). *Islam: A short biography*. New York: Modern Library.

—. (2008). *The bible: A short biography*. New York: Modern Library.

—. (2014). *Fields of blood: Religion and the history of violence*. New York: Knopf.

Arntz, W. (Director); Chasse, B. (Director); Vicente, M. (Director). *What The [bleeb] Do We Know?* [Motion Picture]. USA: Captured Light.

Aslam, M. (2015). "Pakistan." In *Spirit possession around the world: Possession, communion and demon expulsion across cultures*. Ed. J.P. Laycock. Pp. 271-275. Santa Barbara: ABC-CLIO.

Babbin, J. (Producer) & Petrie, D. (Director). (1976). *Sybil* [televised miniseries]. USA: Lorimar.

Baglio, M. (2009). *The rite: The making of a modern exorcist*. New York: Doubleday.

Baird, R. (Producer); Russell, K. (Producer); Solo, R.H. (Producer) & Russell, K. (Director). *The devils* [Motion picture]. France: Warner Brothers.

Balikci, A. (1967). "Shamanistic behavior among the Netsilik Eskimos." In *Magic, witchcraft, & curing*. Ed. J. Middleton. Pp. 191-209. Austin: University of Texas Press.

Bakkevig, J.F., & Sigmund, K. (2010). "Is the diagnostic and statistical manual of mental disorders, fourth edition, histrionic personality

disorder category a valid construct?" *Comprehensive Psychiatry, 51*, 462-470.
Bamberger, J.E. (2006). *Evagruis Ponticus: The praktikos & chapters on prayer*. Collegeville, MN: Cistercian Publications.
Barnes, B.D. (2015). "Incantation bowls." In *Spirit possession around the world: Possession, communion and demon expulsion across cultures*. Ed. J.P. Laycock. Pp. 162-164. Santa Barbara: ABC-CLIO.
Basham, D. (1971). *Can a Christian have a demon?* Kirkwood, MO: Christian Impact Books.
Baxendale, S. (2003). "Epilepsy at the movies: possession to presidential assassination." *Lancet Neurology, 2 (12)*: 764-770.
Bay, M. (Producer) & Douglas, A. (Director). (2005). *The Amityville horror* [Motion Picture]. USA: MGM.
BBC. (2006). "'Witchcraft' study prompts action." Retrieved on March 15, 2015 from: http://news.bbc.co.uk/2/hi/uk_news/5129418.stm.
—. (2009). "BBC Radio 2–The Radcliffe and Maconie Show, 30/11/ 2009". *BBC. 2009-11 30.* Retrieved 2015-04-15.
Beal, E.W. (1978). "Use of the extended family in the treatment of multiple personality". *American Journal of Psychiatry, 135*, 539-542.
Bell, C. (2015a). "Nechung oracle." In *Spirit possession around the world: Possession, communion and demons*. Ed. J.P. Laycock. Pp. 249-251. Santa Barbara: ABC-CLIO.
—. (2015b). "Tibet." In *Spirit possession around the world: Possession, communion and demon expulsion across cultures*. Ed. J.P. Laycock. Pp. 344-349. Santa Barbara: ABC-CLIO.
Bell, T. (1990). *Preventing adolescent relapse: A guide for parents, teachers and counselors*. Independence, MO: Herald/House Independence Press.
Bend, C., & Wiger, T. (1988). *Birth of a modern shaman: A documented journey and guide to personal transformation*. St. Paul, MN: Llewellyn.
Benet, S.V. (1937). *The devil and Daniel Webster*. New York: Farrar and Rinehart.
Benski, T. (Producer); Bronfman, J. (Producer); Columbus, C. (Producer); Columbus, E. (Producer); Godzinskaya, J. (Producer); Johnes, A. (Producer); Mas, S. (Producer); Molnar, L. (Producer); Ochoa, L. (Producer); Sackler, M. (Producer); Sagalchik, A. (Producer); Sant'Anna, L. (Producer); & Eggers (Director). (2015). *The witch* [Motion Picture]. USA: Parts and Labor.
Berger, A.A. (1997). *Postmortem for a postmodernist*. Walnut Creek, CA: AltaMira.
Berman, M. (1981). *The reenchantment of the world*. Cornell: Cornell University Press.

Berne, E. (1964). *Games people play: The basic handbook of transactional analysis*. New York: Ballantine.

Bers, F. (1934). "Like a perpetual sickness"–"Die Gebete nach der hl. Messe", *Theol Prakt. (original article in German) Quartalschrift 87*, 162-163.

Bevan, T. (Producer); Coen, E. (Director) & Coen, J. (Director). (2009). *A serious man* [Motion picture]. USA: Focus.

Beyernstein, B.L. (1995). "Dissociative states: Possession and exorcism." In *The encyclopedia of the paranormal*. Ed. G. Stein. New York: Prometheus.

Birtalan, A. (2015). "Mongolia." In *Spirit possession around the world: Possession, communion and demon expulsion across cultures*. Ed. J.P. Laycock. Pp. 239-242. Santa Barbara: ABC-CLIO.

Bissell, T. (2016). *Apostle: Travels among the tombs of the twelve*. New York: Pantheon.

Blacker, C. (1975). *The catalpa bow: A study in shamanistic practices in Japan*. London: George Allen and Unwin, Ltd.

Blatty, W. (1971). *The exorcist*. New York: Harper and Row.

—. (1974). *William Peter Blatty on 'the exorcist' from novel to film*. New York: Bantam Books.

—. (1981). *Legion*. New York: Tor.

Blatty, W. (Producer) & Friedken, W. (Director). (1973). *The exorcist* [Motion picture]. USA: Warner Brothers.

Blosser, B.P. (2015). "Benedict medal." In *Spirit possession around the world: Possession, communion and demon expulsion across cultures*. Ed. J.P. Laycock. Pp. 37-39. Santa Barbara: ABC-CLIO.

Blumhofer, E.L. (2000). "Charismatic movement." In *Contemporary American religion*. Ed. W.C. Roof. Pp. 108-110. New York: MacMillan.

Boardman, P.H. (Producer); Flynn, B. (Producer) & Derrickson, S. (2005). *The exorcism of Emily Rose* [Motion picture]. USA: Screen Gems.

Boas, F. (1930). *The religion of the Kwakuitl*. New York: Literary Licensing.

Boggs, J.M. (1996). *The art of watching films*. 4th ed. Mountain View, CA: Mayfield.

Boorman, J. (Producer) & Boorman, J. (Director). *The exorcist II: The heretic* [Motion picture]. USA: Warner Brothers.

Borch-Jacobsen, M. (1997). "Sybil: The making of a disease: An interview with Dr. Herbert Spiegel." *New York Review of Books*, *44*, 7. Retrieved on February 5, 2013 from:
http://www.nybooks.com/articles/archives/1997/apr/24/sybil-the-making-of-a-disease/.

Borg, M.J. (1995). *Meeting Jesus again for the first time: The historical Jesus and the heart of contemporary faith.* San Francisco: HarperSanFrancisco.

—. (2001). *Reading the bible again for the first time: Taking the bible seriously but not literally*. San Francisco: HarperSanFrancisco.

Bottoms, B.L., Shaver, P.R., and Goodman, G.S. (1996). "An analysis of ritualistic and religion-related child abuse allegations." *Law and Human Behavior 20 (1)*: 1-34.

Bourguignon, E. (1976). *Possession.* San Francisco: Chandler and Sharp.

Boysen, G.A., & Van Bergen, A. (2013). "A review of published research on adult dissociative identity disorder: 2000-2010." *Journal of Nervous Mental Disorder, 201 (1)*: 5-11.

Braak, C. (2015). "Television." In *Spirit possession around the world: Possession, communion and demon expulsion across cultures*. Ed. J.P. Laycock. Pp. 340-342. Santa Barbara: ABC-CLIO.

Brooks, P. (Producer) and Cornwell, P. (Director). *The haunting in Connecticut* [Motion Picture]. USA: Lionsgate.

Brotherton, R. (2015). *Suspicious minds: Why we believe conspiracy theories*. New York: Bloomsbury.

Brown, D. (2001). *Bury my heart at wounded knee: An Indian history of the American west*. New York: Holt.

Bulletin. (1976). "David's short life filled with pain." *The Bulletin*, November 22, 1976. Retrieved on March 14, 2016 from: https://news.google.com/newspapers?nid=1243&dat=19761122&id=9vtXAAAABAJ&sjid=3fYDAAAAIBAJ&pg=6853,1990721&hl=en.

Burton, N. (2015). *The meaning of madness*. 2nd ed. Exeter: Acheron.

Butler, J. (2015). "Changelings." In *Spirit possession around the world: Possession, communion and demon expulsion across cultures*. Ed. J.P. Laycock. Pp. 68-71. Santa Barbara: ABC-CLIO.

Bradnick, D. (2015). "Deliverance ministry." In *Spirit possession around the world: Possession, communion and demon expulsion across cultures*. Ed. J. P. Laycock. Pp. 104-107. Santa Barbara: ABC-CLIO.

Bredero, A. H. (2001). *Bernard of Clairvaux: Between cult and history*. New York: Eerdmans.

Brendsma, J.M., & Ludwig, A.M. (1974). "A case of multiple personality: Diagnosis and therapy". *International Journal of Clinical and Experiential Hypnosis*, *22*, 216-233.

Brock, R.N., & Parker, R.A. (2008). *Saving paradise: How Christianity traded love of this world for crucifixion and empire*. Boston: Beacon Press.

Brown, K.M. (1991). *Mama Lola: A Vodun priestess in Brooklyn*. Berkeley: University of California Press.
Brown, P. (2015). *Personal communication*. January 22, 2015.
Buber, M. (1970). *I and thou*. Trans. W. Kaufman. New York, Scribner.
Bulgakov, M. (1966, 2008). *The master and margarita*. Trans. by H. Aplin. New York: OneWorld.
Bull, D.L. (2001). "A phenomological model for therapeutic exorcism for dissociative identity disorder." *Journal of Psychology and Theology*, *29*, 131-139.
Bull, D.L., Ellason, J.W. & Ross, C.A. (1998). "Exorcism revisited: Positive outcomes with disassociated identify disorder". *Journal of Psychology and Theology*, *26*, 188-196.
Bultmann, R. (1969). *New testament and mythology*. Minneapolis, MN: Fortress.
Burke, D. (2011). "Demon days: Exorcism is experiencing a renaissance in American Catholicism. The devil is in the details." *Utne*, *167*, 64-67.
Cairns, D. (1960). "Phenomenology" in *Dictionary of philosophy*, Ed. D.D. Runes. Pp. 231-234. New York, Philosophy Library.
Campbell, J. (1979). *The masks of God: Complete four volumes*. New York: Penguin.
Cantero, J.L., Atienza, M., Stickgold, R., Kahana, M.J., Madsen, J.R. & Kocsis, B. (2003). "Sleep dependent theta oscillations in the human hippocampus and neocortex. *Journal of Neuroscience*, *23*, 10897-10903.
Cappucci, J. (2015a). "Ba'al Shem Tov." In *Spirit possession around the world: Possession, communion and demon expulsion across cultures*. Ed. J.P. Laycock. Pp. 27-29. Santa Barbara: ABC-CLIO.
—. (2015b). "Quakerism." In *Spirit possession around the world: Possession, communion and demon expulsion across cultures*. Ed. J.P. Laycock. Pp. 295-297. Santa Barbara: ABC-CLIO.
Cardena, E., & Gleaves, D.H. (2007). "Dissociative disorders." In *Adult psychopathology diagnosis*. 5th edition. Eds. M. Hersen, S.M. Turner, and D.C. Beidel. Hoboken, NJ: Wiley and Sons.
Cardin, M. (2015a). "Daimon." In *Spirit possession around the world: Possession, communion and demon expulsion across cultures*. Ed. J.P. Laycock. Pp. 91-92. Santa Barbara: ABC-CLIO.
Carroll, J. (2002). *Constantine's sword: The church and the Jews*. New York: Mariner.
—. (2014). *Christ actually: The son of God for the secular age*. New York: Viking.
Casey, E. (2004). *The essential Casey*. New York: Penguin.

Cassian, John. (2018). *The conferences of John Cassian*. Trans. C.S. Gibson. Retrieved from http://www.ccel.org/ccel/cassian/conferences.html on April 12, 2018.

Catechism of the Catholic Church. (1997). U.S. Conference of Catholic Bishops. New York: Doubleday.

Catholic Women's League. (2010). "A history of Birmingham archdiocese." Retrieved on February 9, 2016 from: http://www.catholicwomensleague.org/pdfs/CWL%20SUMMER%20PDF.pdf.

Channey, J. (2012). "Nicki Minaj's Grammy performance has angered the Catholic league." *The Washington Post*, February 13, 2012. Retrieved on April 20, 2016 from: https://www.washingtonpost.com/blogs/celebritology/post/nicki-minajs-grammy-performance-has-angered-the-catholic-league/2012/02/13/gIQAfVVfBR_blog.html.

Chaudhuri, S. (2012). "Women as easy scapegoats: Witchcraft accusations and women as targets in tea plantations in India." *Violence Against Women, 18 (10)*: 1213-1234.

Christensen, D. (Producer) & Christensen, D. (Director). (1922). *Häxan: Witchcraft through the Ages* [Motion picture]. Sweden: Aljosha.

Clark, D. (Producer) & Hale, W. (Director). (1983). *The demon murder case* [Motion Picture]. USA: NBC.

Clinebell, C.H. (1976). *Counseling for liberation*. Minneapolis, MN: Fortress.

Cocn, E. (Producer), & Coen, J. (Director). (2000). *O' Brother, Where Art Thou?* [Motion picture]. USA: Touchstone.

Cohen, E. (2002). "The placebo disavowed: Or the unveiling of the bio-medical imagination." *Yale Journal for Humanities in Medicine*. Accessed on November 13, 2012, from: http://yjhm.yale.edu/essays/ecohenprint.htm.

—. (2008). "What is spirit possession? Defining, comparing, and explaining two possession forms." *Ethnos, 73:* 101-26.

Confucius. (trans. 1995). *The analects*. New York: Dover.

Conrad, J. (1902, 1990). *Heart of darkness*. New York: Dover.

Cook, W.R. (2009). *The Catholic church: A history*. Chantilly, VA: The Teaching Company.

Cortes, J.B., & Gatti, F.M. (1975). *The case against possession and exorcism*. New York: Vantage Press.

Cox, H. (1995). *Fire from heaven: The rise of Pentecostal spirituality and the reshaping of religion in the twenty-first century*. Reading, MA: Addison-Wesley.

Crabtree, A. (1988). *Animal magnetism, early hypnotism and psychical research, 1766-1925: An annotated bibliography*. White Plains, NY: Kraus International.

—. (1997a). *Multiple man: Explorations in multiple personality and possession*. New York: St. Martin's Press.

—. (1997b). *Trance Zero: Breaking the spell of conformity*. Toronto: Summerville.

Crapanzano, V., & Garrison, V. (1977). *Case studies in spirit possession*. New York: John Wiley and Sons.

Crisplip, A.T. (2005). *From monastery to hospital: Christian monasticism and the transformation of health care in late antiquity*. Ann Arbor, MI: University of Michigan Press.

Crossan, J.D. (1999). *The Birth of Christianity: Discovering what happened in the years immediately after the execution of Jesus*. New York: HarperOne.

Crow, J.L. (2015). "Spiritualism." In *Spirit possession around the world: Possession, communion and demon expulsion across cultures*. Ed. J.P. Laycock. Pp. 323-328. Santa Barbara: ABC-CLIO.

Csordas, T. (2002). *Body, meaning, healing*. New York: Palgrave.

Cumo, C. (2015). "International association of exorcists." In *Spirit possession around the world: Possession, communion and demon expulsion across cultures*. Ed. J.P. Laycock. Pp. 164-165. Santa Barbara: ABC-CLIO.

—. (2015b). "Psychological interpretations." In *Spirit possession around the world: Possession, communion and demon expulsion across cultures*. Ed. J.P. Laycock. Pp. 291-293. Santa Barbara: ABC-CLIO.

Cuneo, M.W. (1999). *The smoke of Satan*. Baltimore: John Hopkins University Press.

—. (2000). "Exorcism." In *Contemporary American religion*. Ed. W.C. Roof. Pp. 243-245. New York: MacMillan.

—. (2001). *American exorcism: Expelling demons in the land of plenty*. New York: Doubleday.

Dai, B. (1973). "Zen and psychotherapy." In *Religious systems and psychotherapy*. Ed. H.C. Cox. Pp. 132-142. Springfield, IL: Bannerstone House.

Dandelion, B.P. (2008). *Quakers: A very short introduction*. Oxford: Oxford University Press.

Dart, T. (2015). "Bobby Jindal: Republican who brought creationism into schools to enter election." *The Guardian*, Retrieved on June 24, 2015 from: http://www.theguardian.com/usnews/2015/jun/24/bobby-jindal-republicancreationism-2016-election?CMP=ema_565.

Davies, O. (2015). "Lukins, George." In *Spirit possession around the world: Possession, communion and demon expulsion across cultures*. Ed. J.P. Laycock. Pp. 222-224. Santa Barbara: ABC-CLIO.

Davies, S.L. (1995). *Jesus the healer: Possession, trance and the origin of Christianity*. New York: Continuum.

Dawson, A. (2015). "Brazil." In *Spirit possession around the world: Possession, communion and demon expulsion across cultures*. Ed. J.P. Laycock. Pp. 49-52. Santa Barbara: ABC CLIO.

Deeley, Q., Oakley, D.A., Walsh, E., Bell, V., Mehta, M.A., & Halligan, P.W. (2014). "Modelling psychiatric and cultural possession phenomena with suggestion and fMRI." *Cortex*, *53*, 107-119.

De Haven, C. (Producer) & Blatty, W. (Director). *The exorcist III: Legion* [Motion picture]. USA: Morgan Creek.

Delgado, S. (2014). "Outlander slams Christianity: The new Starz series does its part to attack the faith." *National Review*, September 8, 2014. Retrieved on June 23, 2016 from: http://www.nationalreview.com/article/387429/outlander-slams-christianity-j-delgado.

Dennis, G.W. (2015). "Judaism." In *Spirit possession around the world: Possession, communion and demon expulsion across cultures*. Ed. J.P. Laycock. Pp. 190-195. Santa Barbara: ABC-CLIO.

Desmond, J.F. (2014). "Exorcist writer gets response from Holy See on Georgetown petition." *National Catholic Register*. Retrieved on March 23, 2016 from: http://www.ncregister.com/daily-news/holy-see-responds-to-william-peter-blattys-canon law-petition-for-georgetow.

Diamond, S.A. (2011). "Exorcism as psychotherapy: A clinical psychologist examines so-called demonic possession." Retrieved on February 24, 2017 from: https://www.psychologytoday.com/blog/evil-deeds/201102/exorcism-psychotherapyclinical-psychologist-examines-so-called-demonic.

Dien, S., Alexander, M., & Napier, A.D. (2008). "Jinn, psychiatry and contested notions of misfortune among east London Bangladeshis." *Transcultural Psychiatry; 35:* 31-55.

Dein, S., & Samad Illaiee, A. (2009). "Jinn and mental health: Looking at jinn possession in modern psychiatric practice". *Royal College of Psychiatrists, 37 (9)*. Retrieved on March 18, 2015 from: http://pb.rcpsych.org/content/37/9/290.

De Fina, B. (Producer). & Scorsese, M. (Director). *The last temptation of Christ* (Motion picture). USA: Universal.

Demos, J. (2008). *The enemy within: 2,000 years of witch-hunting in the Western world*. New York: Viking.

Deslippe, P. (2015) "Larson, Bob." In *Spirit possession around the world: Possession, communion and demon expulsion across cultures*. Ed. J.P. Laycock. Pp. 211-213. Santa Barbara: ABC-CLIO.

de Tocqueville, A. (2000). *Democracy in America*. San Francisco: Harper Perennial.

Dick, P.K. (2011). *The exegesis of Philip K. Dick*. Eds. P. Jackson & J. Lethan. New York: Houghton Mifflin Harcourt.

Diderot, D. (1796/1974). *The nun*. Trans. L. Tancock. New York: Penguin.

Dolce, L. (2015). "Japan." In *Spirit possession around the world: Possession, communion and demon expulsion across cultures*. Ed. J.P. Laycock. Pp. 178-185. Santa Barbara: ABC-CLIO.

Dollar, N.R. (2015a). "Knight, JZ." In *Spirit possession around the world: Possession, communion and demon expulsion across cultures*. Ed. J.P. Laycock. Pp. 205-207. Santa Barbara: ABC-CLIO.

—. (2015b). "Wickland, Carl." In *Spirit possession around the world: Possession, communion and demons*. Ed. J.P. Laycock. Pp. 371. Santa Barbara: ABC-CLIO.

Donnelly, N.D. (1994). *Changing lives of refugee Hmong women*. Seattle: University of Washington Press.

Dossey, L. (2003). "Forward" in *Coyote Healing: Miracles in native healing*. L. Mehl-Madrona. Rochester, VT: Bear & Co.

Dostoevsky, F. (1872, 2009). *The devils* (*The possessed*). New York: EZ Readers.

DuBois, T.A. (2009). *An introduction to shamanism*. New York: Cambridge University Press.

Duppils, S. (2015a). "Gastkramad." In *Spirit possession around the world: Possession, communion and demon expulsion across cultures*. Ed. J.P. Laycock. Pp. 129. Santa Barbara: ABC-CLIO.

—. (2015b). "Ghost sickness." In *Spirit possession around the world: Possession, communion and demon expulsion across cultures*. Ed. J.P. Laycock. Pp. 136. Santa Barbara: ABC-CLIO.

—. (2015c.) "Possessed objects." In *Spirit possession around the world: Possession, communion and demon expulsion across cultures*. Ed. J.P. Laycock. Pp. 286-288. Santa Barbara: ABC-CLIO.

During, E.H., Elahi, F.M., Moro, M.R., & Baubet, T. (2011). "A critical review of dissociative trance and possession disorders: Etiological, diagnostic, therapeutic and nosological issues." *Canadian Journal of Psychiatry, 56 (4)*: 235-242.

Dziegielewski, S. (2010). *DSM-IV-TR in action*. Second edition. Hoboken, NJ: Wiley.

Eco, U. (2007). *Foucault's pendulum*. New York: Mariner.

—. (2011). *The Prague cemetery*. New York: Mariner.
Economist. (2011). "How Luther went viral: Five centuries before Facebook and the Arab spring, social media helped bring about the Reformation." *401*: 93-96.
—. (2012a). "China and the paradox of prosperity." *492*: 9.
—. (2012b). "Toil and trouble: In a corner of north-eastern India, old superstitions die hard." *492*: 48.
Egan, C. (2013). "The derivative works of Robert Louis Stevenson." Retrieved on February 5, 2013 from: http://www.robert-louis-stevenson.org/derivative-works.
Ehrenreich, B. (2009). *Bright-sided: How the relentless promotion of positive thinking is undermining America*. New York: Metropolitan.
Ehrman, B. (2005). *Lost Christianities: The battle for scriptures and faiths we never knew*. Oxford: Oxford University Press.
—. (2014). *How Jesus became God: The exaltation of a Jewish preacher from Galilee*. New York: HarperOne.
Elby, T. (2015a). "Tantra." In *Spirit possession around the world: Possession, communion and demon expulsion across cultures*. Ed. J.P. Laycock. Pp. 335-337. Santa Barbara: ABC-CLIO.
—. (2015). "Teyyam." In *Spirit possession around the world: Possession, communion and demon expulsion across cultures*. Ed. J.P. Laycock. Pp. 342-344. Santa Barbara: ABC-CLIO.
Eliade, M. (trans. 1982). *A history of religious ideas: From Guatama Buddha to the triumph of Christianity. Vol. 2*. Chicago: University of Chicago Press.
Ellenberger, H.F. (1970). *Discovery of the unconscious*. New York: Basic Books.
Elliot, T.S. (1991). *Collected Poems: 1909-1962*. New York: Harcourt Brace Jovanovich.
Eneborg, Y.M. (2015). "Islam." In *Spirit possession around the world: Possession, communion and demon expulsion across cultures*. Ed. J.P. Laycock. Pp. 166-171. Santa Barbara: ABC-CLIO.
Engler, S. (2015). "Kardecism." In *Spirit possession around the world: Possession, communion and demon expulsion across cultures*. Ed. J.P. Laycock. Pp. 198-202. Santa Barbara: ABC-CLIO.
Eron, J.B., & Lund, T.W. (1996). *Narrative solutions in brief therapy*. New York: Guilford.
Espí Forcén, C., & Espí Forcén, F. (2014). "Demonic possessions and mental illness: Discussion of selected cases in late medieval hagiographical literature." *Early Science and Medicine*, *19* (*3*): 258-279.

Evans, D. (1971). *Tommy Johnson*. Littlehampton: Littlehampton Book Service.

Ezzy, D. (2015). Paganism and witchcraft, contemporary." In *Spirit possession around the world: Possession, communion and demon expulsion across cultures*. Ed. J.P. Laycock. Pp. 269-271. Santa Barbara: ABC-CLIO.

Fadiman, A. (1997). *The spirit catches you and you fall down: A Hmong child, her American doctors, and the clash of two cultures*. New York: Farrar, Strauss and Giroux.

Falsh, C. (Producer) & Akselsen, F.H. (Director). (2012). *The exorcist in the 21st century* [Motion picture]. Norway: Nordic World.

"Father Tom". (2015). *Personal communication*. January 17, 2015.

Ferracuti, S., Sacco, R., & Lazzari, R. (1996). "Dissociative trance disorder: clinical and Rorschach findings in ten persons reporting demon possession and treated by exorcism." *Journal of Personality Assessment, 66 (3)*: 525-539.

Field, M.J. (1955). "Witchcraft as a primitive interpretation of mental disorder." *Journal of Mental Science, 101*, 826-833.

Fibiger, M.Q. (2015). "Hinduism." In *Spirit possession around the world: Possession, communion and demon expulsion across cultures*. Ed. J.P. Laycock. Pp. 143-150. Santa Barbara: ABC-CLIO.

Flood, A. (2016). "Fairytales much older than thought, says researchers." *The Guardian*. Retrieved on January 21, 2016 from: http://www.theguardian.com/books/2016/jan/20/fairytales-much-older-than-previously-thought-say-researchers?utm_source=esp&utm_medium=Email&utm_campaign=GU+Today+USA+-+Version+A&utm_term=152229&subid=14329163&CMP=ema_565a.

Floyd, E.R. (1999). *The good, the bad, and the mad: Some weird people in American history*. New York: Fall River Press.

Flynn, B. (Producer) & Håfström, M. (Director). (2011). *The rite* [Motion picture]. USA: New Line.

Foote, B., Smolin, Y., Kaplan, M., Legatt, M.E., Lipschitz, D., (2006). "Prevalence of dissociative disorders among psychiatric patients." *American Journal of Psychiatry, 163 (4)*; 623-9.

Foote, B., Smolin, Y., Neft, D.L., & Lipschitz, D. (2008). "Dissociative disorders and suicidality in outpatient patients." *Journal of Nervous and Mental Disease, 196, (1)*: 29-36.

Foster, D. K. (2008). "An interview with Francis and Judith McNutt". Retrieved from http://www.masteringlife.org/index.php/mastering-life/articles/miscellaneous/item/35-interview-francis-judith-macnutt on January 26, 2016.

Foucault, M. (1961, trans. 1973). *Madness & civilization: A history of insanity in an age of reason*. New York: Vintage.
—. (1966, trans. 1973). *The order of things: An archaeology of the human sciences*. New York: Vintage.
Fox, J.R. (1967). "Witchcraft and clanship in Cochiti therapy." In *Magic, witchcraft & curing*. Ed. J. Middleton. Pp. 255-284. Austin: University of Texas Press.
Frankl, V. E. (1969, 1988). *The will to meaning: Foundations and applications of logotherapy*. New York: Meridian.
Frattaroli, E. (2001). *Healing the soul in the age of the brain: Why medication isn't enough*. New York: Penguin.
Freed, S.A., & Freed, R.S. (1976). "Spirit possession as illness in a north Indian village". In *Magic, witchcraft and curing*. Ed. J. Middleton. Austin, TX: University of Texas Press.
Freeman, R. (2003). "The teyyam tradition of Kerala." In *The Blackwell Companion to Hinduism*. Ed. G. Flood. Pp. 307-326. Oxford: Blackwell.
Freud, S. (1923). "A seventeenth-century demonological neurosis." *The standard edition of the complete works of Sigmund Freud XIX*. Pp. 72-105. London: The Hogarth Press.
Gabel, P. (2013). *Another way of seeing: Essays on transforming law, politics and culture*. New Orleans, Quid Pro Books.
Gallop. (2005). http://www.gallup.com/poll/17275/OneThird-Americans-Believe-Dearly-May-Departed.aspx?g_source=ghosts&g_medium=search&g_campaign=tiles. Retrieved on September 26, 2016.
—. (2015). , 2015.
Ganaway, G. (1989). "Historical versus narrative truth: Clarifying the role of exogenous trauma in the etiology of MPD and its variants." *Dissociation, 2:* 205-220.
Garcia, C. (1993). *Dreaming in Cuban*. New York: Ballantine.
Gast, U., Rodewald, F., Nickel, V., & Emrich, H.M. (2001). "Prevalence of dissociative disorders among psychiatric inpatients in a German university clinic." *Journal of Nervous and Mental Disease, 189 (4)*: 249-257.
Gazzaniga, M.S. (2011). *Who's in charge? Free will and the science of the brain*. New York: Ecco.
Gerard, R. (1979). *The scapegoat*. Baltimore: John Hopkins University Press.
—. (1989). *Violence and the sacred*. Baltimore: John Hopkins University Press.
Germiniani, F.M., Miranda, A.P., Ferenczy, P., Munhoz, R.P., & Teive, H.A. (2012). "Tourette's syndrome: from demonic possession and

psychoanalysis to the discovery of genes." *Arquivos de neuro-psiquiatria, 70 (7)*: 547-540.

Gettis, A. (1976). "Psychotherapy as exorcism." *Journal of Religion and Health, 15 3*: 188-190.

Gibson, M. (2006). *Possession, Puritanism and Print: Darrell, Harsnett, Shakespeare and the Elizabethan Exorcism Controversy*. London: Pickering and Chatto.

Ginzburg, K., Somer, E., Tamarkin, G., & Kramer, L. (2010). "Clandestine psychopathology: Unrecognized dissociative disorders in inpatient psychiatry." *Journal of Nervous and Mental Disorders, 198 (5)*: 378-381.

Goethe, J.W.V. (1808, 1832, 1962). *Faust*. Trans. W. Kaufmann. New York: Anchor.

Golding, W. (1971). *The inheritors*. New York: Pocket Books.

Gomez, L. (2017). *Personal communication*, February 14, 2017.

Gomm, R. (1975). "Bargaining from weakness: Spirit possession on the south Kenya coast. *Man, 10 4*: 504-543.

Good, B. (1994). *Medicine, rationality, and experience: An anthropological perspective*. Cambridge: Cambridge University Press.

Goodman, F. (1981). *The exorcism of Anneliese Michel*. New York: Doubleday.

—. (1988a). *Ecstasy, ritual and alternate reality: Religion in a pluralistic world*. Bloomington: Indiana University Press.

—. (1988b). *How about demons? Possession and exorcism in the modern world*. Bloomington: Indiana University Press.

Gordon, S. (Producer) & Meyer, R. (Director). (2003). *Searching for Haizmann* [Motion Picture]. USA: Centre Communications.

Gottlieb, A. (2012). "Neurons v. free will: The notion of a rational self is under attack again, this time from the march of neuroscience." *Intelligent Life*, 6-7.

Grady, J.L. (undated). "The priest with healing hands: Heroes of the faith." Retrieved on May 27, 2015 from: http://www.charismamag.com/life/351-j15/features/heroes-of-the-faith/1269-the-priest-with-healing-hands.

Graf, S. (2010). *Holotropic breathwork: A new approach to self-exploration and therapy*. New York: SUNY Press.

Graves, G.B. (1988). "Observations on the claims of iatrogenesis on the promulgation of MPD: A discussion." *Dissociation*, *2*, 99-104.

Graves, T. (2008). *Crossroads: The life and afterlife of blues legend Robert Johnson*. New York: Demers.

Greenblatt, S. (1988). *Shakespearean negotiations: The circulation of social energy in Renaissance England*. Berkley: University of California Press.

—. (2011). *The swerve: How the world became modern*. New York: Norton.

Greer, G.L. (2015). "Daoism." In *Spirit possession around the world: Possession, communion and demon expulsion across cultures*. Ed. J.P. Laycock. Pp. 95-97. Santa Barbara: ABC-CLIO.

Grey, J.G. (1959). *The warriors: Reflections of men in battle*. New York: Bison.

Griffin, D.R. (2000). *Reenchantment without supernaturalism: A process philosophy*. Cornell: Cornell University Press.

Groeschel, B.J. (1999). "Forward to the American edition." In *An exorcist tells his story*. Ed. G. Amarth. San Francisco: Ignatius Press.

Guardian. (2008). "The beast within." Originally published December 12, 2008. Retrieved on February 5, 2013 from: http://www.guardian.co.uk/books/2008/dec/13/dr-jekyll-mr-hyde-stevenson.

Guiley, R. (2009). *The encyclopedia of demons and demonology*. New York: Facts on File.

Guralnick, P. (1998). *Searching for Robert Johnson: The Life and Legend of the "King of the Delta Blues Singers"*. New York: Plume.

Halbertal, M. (2012). "Alive and well: Judaism and the Jews." *The Economist, 404*: 8795.

Hale, J.R. (2009). *Exploring the roots of religion*. Chantilly, VA: The Teaching Company.

Halifax, J., & Weidman, H.H. (1973). "Religion as a mediating institution in acculturation." In *Religious systems and psychotherapy*. Springfield, IL: Charles C. Thomas Publishing.

Halliburton, M. (2010). "'Just some spirits': The erosion of spirit possession and the rise of 'tension' in South India." *Culture, Medicine and Psychiatry, 34 (2)*: 380-400.

Hammond, F., & Hammond, I.M. (1973). *Pigs in the parlor: A practical guide to deliverance*. Kirkwood, MO: Impact Christian Books.

Hanley, J., & Brown, A. (2014). "Cultural variations in interpretation of postnatal illness: Jinn possession amongst Muslim communities." *Community Mental Health Journal, 50 (3)*: 348-353.

Hardtke, T. (2015a). "Deaths resulting from exorcisms." In *Spirit possession around the world: Possession, communion and demons*. Ed. J.P. Laycock. Pp. 99-103. Santa Barbara: ABC-CLIO.

—. (2015b). "Menghi, Girolamo." In *Spirit possession around the world: Possession, communion and demon expulsion across cultures*. Ed. J.P. Laycock. Pp. 229-231. Santa Barbara: ABC-CLIO.

Hardy, G. (2014). *Sacred texts of the world*. Chantilly, VA: The Great Courses.

Harland, P. (1999). "Possession and desire: A deconstructivist approach to understanding and working with addictions." Retrieved on October 29, 2014 from: http://www.cleanlanguage.com/addict-I.html.

Harner, M. (1980). *The way of the shaman: A guide to power and healing*. New York: Bantam.

Harris, R. (1999). *Lourdes*. London: Penguin.

Harrison, M.F. (2000). "African-American religions." In *Contemporary American religion*. Ed. W.C. Roof. Pp. 5-9. New York: MacMillan.

Harvey, D. (1989). *The condition of postmodernity*. Oxford: Basil Blackwell.

Harvey, G. (2015). "Shamanism." In *Spirit possession around the world: Possession, communion and demon expulsion across cultures*. Ed. J.P. Laycock. Pp. 86-87. Santa Barbara: ABC-CLIO.

Hatchman, L. (2015). "Conversion disorder." In *Spirit possession around the world: Possession, communion and demon expulsion across cultures*. Ed. J.P. Laycock. Pp. 86-87. Santa Barbara: ABC-CLIO.

Hause, Steven C. (1989). "Anti-Protestant Rhetoric in the Early Third Republic". *French Historical Studies 16 (1)*: 192.

Hayward, R. (2015). "Penn-Lewis, Jessie." In *Spirit possession around the world: Possession, communion and demon expulsion across cultures*. Ed. J.P. Laycock. Pp. 276-278. Santa Barbara: ABC-CLIO.

Hegel, G.W.F. (1968). *Lectures on the philosophy of religion: Together with a work on the proofs of the existence of God*. Trans. Rev. E. B. Speirs, B. D. and J. Burdon Sanderson. 3 volumes. New York: Humanities Press, Inc.

Hegeman, E. (2013). "Ethnic syndromes as disguise for protest against colonialism: Three ethnographic examples." *Journal of Trauma and Dissociation, 14 (2)*: 138-146.

Heidegger, M. (1927, 1962). *Being and time*. New York: Harper & Row.

Helmouth, L. (2014). "Witness to an exorcism: How Pope Francis and the Vatican deal with the devil." Retrieved on October 29, 2014 from: http://www.slate.com/articles/life/faithbased/2014/05/exorcism_in_catholic_church_pop francis_says_satan_the_devil_is_real.1.html.

Herskovits, M.J. (1971). *Life in a Haitian valley*. Garden City, NJ: Doubleday.

Heckman, J. (2015). *Personal communication*. January 16, 2015.

Hillman, J. (1991). *A blue fire: James Hillman reader*. Ed. T. Moore. New York: HarperOne.

Homer. (1999). *The iliad and the odyssey*. Trans. R. Fowles. New York: Penguin.

Hopper, K., & Wanderling, J. (2000). "Revisiting the developed versus developing country distinction in course and outcome in schizophrenia: Results from Isos, the WHO collaborative follow-up project." *Schizophrenia Bulletin*, *26 (4)*, 835.

Hoyerson, J.G. (1996). "Possessed! Some historical, psychiatric and current moments of demonic possession (in Norwegian). *Tidsskr Nor Laegeforen*, *116*: 3602-6.

Houdini, H. (1924/2011). *A magician among the spirits*. Cambridge: Cambridge University Press.

Hoyt, O. (1978). *Exorcism*. New York: Franklin Watts.

Hunter, J.D. (1992). *Culture wars*: *The struggle to control the family, art, education, law and politics in America*. New York: Basic.

Hurston, Z.N. (1938). *Tell my horse*: *Voodoo and life in Haiti and Jamaica*. New York: Harper.

Husserl, E. (1900). *Logical investigations*. New York: Humanities Press.

Huxley, A. (1958). *Ape and Essence*. New York: Bantam.

—. (1971). *The devils of Loudun*. New York: HarperPerennial.

ICD10data.com. (2013). The free medical coding reference. Retrieved on February 12, 2013 from: http://www.icd10data.com/ICD10CM/Codes/F01-F99/F40-F48/F44/F44.89.

Igreja, V., Dias-Lambranca, B., Hershey, D.A., Racin, L., Richters, A., & Reis, R. (2010). "The epidemiology of spirit possession in the aftermath of mass political violence in Mozambique." *Social Science Medicine*, *71 (3)*: 592-599.

Illich, I. (1982). *Medical nemesis*: *The expropriation of health*. New York: Pantheon.

International Catholic Charismatic Renewal Services. (2007). *Guidelines on prayers for healing*. Ferryville, MI: Vera Cruz Publications.

Internet Movie Database. Search for the word "exorcism" done on January 26, 2013.

Irmak, M.K. (2014). "Schizophrenia or possession?" *Journal of Religion and Health*, *53 (3)*: 773-777.

Irving, *W*. (1824, 1998). *Complete tales of Washington Irving*. New York: Da Capo.

Isaacs, C. (2010). *Revelations and possession*: *Distinguishing spiritual from psychological experiences*. New York: Morris.

Islam, F., & Campbell, R.A. (2014). "'Satan has afflicted me!' Jinn possession and mental illness in the Quran." *Journal of Religion and Health, 53 (1)*: 229-43.

Ivey, A. E., D'Andrea, M.J., & Ivey, M.B. (2012). *Theories of counseling and psychotherapy: A multicultural perspective*. Thousand Oaks, CA: Sage.

Jackson, S. (1954). *The bird's nest*. New York: Farrar, Strauss and Young.

Jacob. (2013). "Missionaries and exorcisms." Retrieved on March 8, 2017 from: https://bycommonconsent.com/2013/04/18/missionaries-and-exorcisms/#more-44342.

Jacob, F. (2015a). "Delphic oracle." In *Spirit possession around the world: Possession, communion and demon expulsion across cultures*. Ed. J.P. Laycock. Pp. 107-109. Santa Barbara: ABC-CLIO.

—. (2015b). "Jinn." In *Spirit possession around the world: Possession, communion and demon expulsion across cultures*. Ed. J.P. Laycock. Pp. 187-188. Santa Barbara: ABC-CLIO.

Jacobs, A. (2005). *The Narnian: The life and imagination of C.S. Lewis*. San Francisco: Harper.

Jacobs, A.J. (2012). *Drop dead healthy: One man's humble quest for bodily perfection*. New York: Simon and Schuster.

James, G. (1995). *Interpreting Religion: The Phenomenological Approaches of Pierre Daniël Chantepie de la Saussaye, W. Brede Kristensen, and Gerardus van der Leeuw*. Washington: Catholic University of America Press.

James, K. (1597/2016). *Daemonologie. A Critical Edition*. CreateSpace Independent Publishing.

James, W. (1902/2011). *Varieties of religious experiences: A study in human nature*. Oxford: Oxford World's Classics.

Joannes Paules PPII. (1995). *Evangelium Vitae*. Retrieved on October 24, 2014 from: http://www.vatican.va/holy_father/john_paul_ii/encyclicals/documents/hf_jp ii_enc_25031995_evangelium-vitae_en.html.

Josephus, F. (2001). *Antiquities*. Trans. W. Whiston. Retrieved from: http://www.josephus.org/ on January 27, 2016.

John, C. (2005b). "Exorcisms are part of our culture." Retrieved on March 12, 2015 from: http://news.bbc.co.uk/2/hi/uk_news/4596127.stm.

Johnson, J. (2010). *Alcoholism, wrongly diagnosed: The real reason why it is so hard to break the cycle of alcoholism & drug addiction, and how to win, with God's help*. Los Angeles: Triumph.

Johnson, L.T. (2008). *Mystical traditions: Judaism, Christianity and Islam*. Chantilly, VA: The Teaching Company.

Johnson, N. (Producer) & Johnson, N. (Director). (1957). *The three faces of Eve* [Motion picture]. USA: 20th Century Fox.

Jong, J.D., & Ries, R. (2013). "Collective trauma processing: dissociation as a way of processing postwar traumatic stress in Guinea Bissau." *Transcultural Psychiatry, 50 (5)*: 644-661.

Jongsma, A.E., & Peterson, M. (2006). *The complete adult psychotherapy treatment planner*. 4th ed. Hoboken, NJ: Wiley.

Jung, C.G. (1968). *Man and his symbols*. New York: Dell.

—. (1976). *The portable Jung*. New York: Penguin.

Haar, B.J.T. (2015). "China." In *Spirit possession around the world: Possession, communion and demon expulsion across cultures*. Ed. J.P. Laycock. Pp. 76-80. Santa Barbara: ABC-CLIO.

Kaiser, R.B. (2002). *Clerical error: A true story*. New York: Continuum.

Kallendorf, H. (2003). *Exorcism and its texts: Subjectivity in early modern literature of England and Spain*. Toronto: University of Toronto Press.

Kaplan, M. (2012). *The science of monsters: The origins of the creatures we love to fear*. New York: Scribner.

Karlsson, E. (2014a). "Schizophrenia is not demonic possession". From http://debunkingdenialism.com/tag/m-kemal-irmak/. Retrieved on January 2, 2015.

—. (2014b). "Mailbag: Faith healing for schizophrenia is a bad idea". Retrieved on January 2, 2015 from: http://debunkingdenialism.com/2014/12/26/mailbag-faith-healing-for-schizophrenia-is-a-bad-idea/.

Kazantzakis, N. (1980). *The last temptation of Christ*. Trans. P.A. Bien. New York: Touchstone.

Keeney, B.P. (1996). *Everyday soul: Awakening the spirit in daily life*. New York: Riverhead.

—. (2003). *Ropes to God: Experiencing the Bushman spiritual universe*. Philadelphia: Ringing Rocks Press.

Kehoe, A.B. (2000). *Shamans and religion: An anthropological exploration in critical thinking*. Prospect Heights: Waveland Press.

Kelly, S., & Rogers, R. (1993). *Saints preserve us: Everything you need to know about every saint you'll ever need*. New York: Random House.

Kemp, S., & Williams, K. (1987). "Demonic possession and mental disorder in medieval and early modern Europe." *Psychological Medicine, 17 (1)*: 21-29.

Keyes, D. (1966). *Flowers for Algernon*. New York: Harcourt Brace.

—. (1981). *The minds of Billy Milligan*. New York: Random House.

Khalifa, N., & Hardie, T. (2005). "Possession and jinn." *Journal of the Royal Society of Medicine, 98:* 351-3.

Khan, I.D., & Sahni, A.K. (2013). "Possession syndrome at high altitude (4575 m/15000 ft.)." *Kathmandu University Medical Journal, 11 (43)*: 253-5.

Kiely, D.M., & McKenna, C. (2007). *The dark sacrament*: *True stories of modern-day demon possession and exorcism*. New York: HarperOne.

Kiev, A. (1966). "Psychotherapeutic value of spirit-possession." In *Trance and possession states*. Ed. R. Prince. Montreal: R.M. Bucke Memorial Society.

—. (1969). "Primitive religious rites and behavior: Clinical considerations." In *Clinical psychiatry and religion*. Ed. E.M. Patterson. Pp. 119-131. New York: Little, Brown.

—. (1972). *Transcultural psychiatry*. New York: Free Press.

—. (1973). "Magic, faith and healing in modern psychiatry." In *Religious systems and psychotherapy*. Ed. H.C. Cox. Pp. 225-235. Springfield, IL: Bannerstone House.

Kirby, A. (2006). "The death of postmodernism and beyond." *Philosophy Now*, *58*. Retrieved on February 19, 2016 from: https://philosophynow.org/issues/58/The_Death_of_Postmodernism_And_Beyond.

Kleinman, A. (1981). *Patients and healers in the context of culture*: *An exploration of the borderland between anthropology, medicine and psychiatry*. Berkeley: University of California.

Knight, K. (2012). "Medal of St. Benedict." *New Advent* website. Retrieved on February 3, 2016 from: http://www.newadvent.org/cathen/13338a.htm.

Koning, N. (2013). "Witchcraft beliefs and witch hunts: An interdisciplinary explanation." *Human Nature*, *24 (2)*: 158-181.

Koningisor, C. (2011). "The return of the Catholic exorcism." *The Atlantic*. January 27, 2011. Retrieved on November 1, 2016 from: http://www.theatlantic.com/national/archive/2011/01/the-return-of-the-catholic-exorcism/70364/.

Kottler, J.A. (2003). *On being a therapist. 3rd ed.* San Francisco: Jossey-Bass.

Kugel, J.L. (2011). *In the valley of the shadow*: *On the foundations of religious belief (and their connection to a certain, fleeting state of mind.)* New York: Free Press.

Kuhn, T. (1962). *The structure of scientific revolution*. Chicago, IL: University of Chicago Press.

Kung, H. (1987, trans. 1988). *Theology for the third millennium: An ecumenical view*. New York: Doubleday.
Kustron, K.G. (2015). "Holy water." In *Spirit possession around the world: Possession, communion and demon expulsion across cultures*. Ed. J.P. Laycock. Pp. 154-155. Santa Barbara: ABC-CLIO.
Kutchins, H., & Kirk, S.A. (2003). *Making us crazy: DSM, the psychiatric bible and the creation of mental disorders*. New York: Free Press.
Kraft, C.H. (1997). *I give you authority*. Grand Rapids, MI: Chosen Books.
—. (2010). *Two hours to freedom: A simple and effective method for healing and deliverance*. Grand Rapids, MI: Chosen Books.
Labous, J. (2015). "The traditional mystics going online. *BBC Magazine*. 16 March. Retrieved on May 9, 2016 from: http://www.bbc.com/news/magazine-31859284.
Lambo, T.A. (1956). "Neuropsychiatric observation in the western region of Nigeria". *British Medical Journal*, *2*, 1388-1394.
Lampe, G.W.H. (1972). "The Holy Spirit and the Person of Christ". In *Christ, faith and history: Cambridge studies in Christology*. Eds. S.W. Sykes & J.P. Clayton. Pp. 117-118. Cambridge: Cambridge University Press.
Lancaster, E. (1958). *The final face of Eve*. New York: McGraw-Hill.
Langston, B. (2015). "The boy of Bilston: A strange and long forgotten case of Staffordshire demons." Retrieved on February 8, 2016 from: http://hubpages.com/religion-philosophy/The-Strange-Case-of-The-Boy-of-Bilston.
Laubscher, B.J.F. (1937). *Custom and psychotherapy*. London: Routledge.
Lawson, J. (2015). *Furiously happy: A funny book about horrible things*. New York: Flatiron Press.
Laycock, J.P. (2015a). "Amorth, Gabriele." In *Spirit possession around the world: Possession, communion and demon expulsion across cultures*. Ed. J.P. Laycock. Pp. 9-10. Santa Barbara: ABC-CLIO.
—. (2015b). "Dancing mania." In *Spirit possession around the world: Possession, communion and demon expulsion across cultures*. Ed. J.P. Laycock. Pp. 92-94. Santa Barbara: ABC-CLIO.
—. (2015c). "Ergotism." In *Spirit possession around the world: Possession, communion and demon expulsion across cultures*. Ed. J.P. Laycock. Pp. 117-118. Santa Barbara: ABC-CLIO.
—. (2015d). "Gay exorcism." In *Spirit possession around the world: Possession, communion and demon expulsion across cultures*. Ed. J.P. Laycock. Pp. 131-132. Santa Barbara: ABC-CLIO.

—. (2015e). "Pigs in the parlor." In *Spirit possession around the world: Possession, communion and demon expulsion across cultures*. Ed. J.P. Laycock. Pp. 285-286. Santa Barbara: ABC-CLIO.

—. (2015f). "Progressive politics." In *Spirit possession around the world: Possession, communion and demon expulsion across cultures*. Ed. J.P. Laycock. Pp. 288-289. Santa Barbara: ABC-CLIO.

Lea, D. (2015). "Dugdale, Richard." In *Spirit possession around the world: Possession, communion and demon expulsion across cultures*. Ed. J.P. Laycock. Pp. 113-114. Santa Barbara: ABC-CLIO.

Leo XIII, P. (1884). *Humanum genus*. Retrieved on October 31, 2014 from: http://www.vatican.va/holy_father/leo_xiii/encyclicals/documents/hf_l-xiii_enc_18840420_humanum-genus_en.html.

—. (1891). *Rerum novarum*. Retrieved on October 31, 2014 from: http://www.vatican.va/holy_father/leo_xiii/encyclicals/documents/hf_l-xiii_enc_15051891_rerum-novarum_en.html.

Leon, L.D. (2000). "Ecstasy." In *Contemporary American religion*. Ed. W.C. Roof. Pp. 213-215. New York: MacMillan.

Lerer, S. (2008). *The history of the English language, 2nd ed*. Chantilly, VA: The Teaching Company.

Levack, B.P. (2013). *The devil within: Possession and exorcism in the Christian west*. New Haven: Yale University Press.

Levenkron, S. (1998). *Cutting: Understanding and overcoming mutilation*. New York: Norton.

Levi-Strauss, C. (1967). "The sorcerer and his magic." In *Magic, witchcraft, &curing*. Ed. J. Middleton. Pp. 23-42. Austin: University of Texas Press.

—. (1968). *The savage mind: Nature of human society*. Chicago: University of Chicago Press.

Lewis, B. (2003). *What went wrong? The clash between Islam and modernity in the Middle East*. San Francisco: Harper Perennial.

Lewis, C.S. (1946). *The screwtape letters*. London: Collins Fontana.

Lewis, I.M. (1989). *Religion in context: Cults and charisma*. Cambridge: Cambridge University Press.

—. (1986/2003). *Ecstatic religion: A study in shamanism and spirit possession*. London: Routledge.

Lewis, S. (2015a). "Bali." In *Spirit possession around the world: Possession, communion and demon expulsion across cultures*. Ed. J.P. Laycock. Pp. 30-32. Santa Barbara: ABC-CLIO.

—. (2015b). "Dissociative identity disorder." *Spirit possession around the world: Possession, communion and demon expulsion across cultures*. Ed. J.P. Laycock. Pp. 111-113. Santa Barbara: ABC-CLIO

Lewis-Fernandez, R., Gorritz, M., Raggio, G.A., Pelaez, C., Chen, H., & Guarnaccia, P.A. (2010). "Association of trauma-related disorders and dissociation with four idioms of distress among Latino psychiatric outpatients." *Culture, Medicine & Psychiatry*, *34 (2)*: 219-243.

Linde, P. (2001). *Of spirits and madness: An American psychiatrist in Africa*. New York: McGraw-Hill.

Linehan. M. (1993). *Skills Training Manual for Treating Borderline Personality Disorder*. New York: Guilford.

Lior, Y. (2015a). "Dybbuk." In *Spirit possession around the world*: *Possession, communion and demon expulsion across cultures*. Ed. J.P. Laycock. Pp. 115-116. Santa Barbara: ABC-CLIO.

Lio, Y. (2015b). "Ibbur." In *Spirit possession around the world*: *Possession, communion and demon expulsion across cultures*. Ed. J.P. Laycock. Pp. 161. Santa Barbara: ABC-CLIO.

Lloyd, S. (2015a). "Ethiopia." In *Spirit possession around the world*: *Possession, communion and demon expulsion across cultures*. Ed. J.P. Laycock. Pp. 119-121. Santa Barbara: ABC-CLIO.

—. (2015b). "Kenya." In *Spirit possession around the world*: *Possession, communion and demon expulsion across cultures*. Ed. J.P. Laycock. Pp. 202-205. Santa Barbara: ABC-CLIO.

—. (2015c). "South Africa." In *Spirit possession around the world*: *Possession, communion and demon expulsion across cultures*. Ed. J.P. Laycock. Pp. 321-323. Santa Barbara: ABC-CLIO.

Loftus, E., & Ketcham, K. (1994). *The myth of repressed memory*: *False memories and allegations of sexual abuse*. New York: St. Martin's Griffith.

Lowe, D. (1972). "Intentionality and the method of history." In *Phenomenology and the social sciences*. Ed. M. Natanson. Evanston, IL: Northwestern University Press.

Lund, H. (2014). *Spirituality, religion and faith in psychotherapy practice*: *Evidence-based expressive methods for mind, brain and body*. New York: Lyceum Books.

Luhrmann, T. (2005). "The art of hearing God: Absorption, dissociation, and contemporary American spirituality." *Spiritus*, *5*: 133-157.

Luhrmann, T.M., Nusbaum, H., & Thisted, R. (2010). "The absorption hypothesis: Learning to hear God in evangelical Christianity." *American Anthropologist*, *12, 1*: 66-78.

Lyotard, J-F. (1997). *The postmodern condition*: *A report on knowledge*. Minneapolis: University of Minnesota Press.

MacLeod, D. (2015a). "Exorcist, The." In *Spirit possession around the world: Possession, communion and demon expulsion across cultures*. Ed. J.P. Laycock. Pp. 121-123. Santa Barbara: ABC-CLIO.
—. (2015b). "Film." In *Spirit possession around the world: Possession, communion and demon expulsion across cultures*. Ed. J.P. Laycock. Pp. 125-127. Santa Barbara: ABC-CLIO.
Mahoney, M. (Producer) & Sargent, J. (Director). (2007). *Sybil* [Televised miniseries]. USA: Warner Brothers.
Malik, K. (2014). *The quest for a moral compass: A global history of ethics*. Brooklyn, NY: Melville.
Mansen, F.D. (2015). "Bentresh stela, the." In *Spirit possession around the world: Possession, communion and demon expulsion across cultures*. Ed. J.P. Laycock. Pp. 39-40. Santa Barbara: ABC-CLIO.
Markis, G.P. (2000). *Changing masters: Spirit possession and identity construction among slave descendants and other subordinates in the Sudan*. Evanston, IL: Northwestern.
Marsden, G.M. (1997). *The outrageous idea of Christian scholarship*. Oxford: Oxford University Press.
Marquez, G.G. (1995). *Of love and other demons*. New York: Knopf.
Mastin, L. (2009). "North Berwick witch trials." Retrieved on November 1, 2016 from: http://www.witchcraftandwitches.com/trials_north_berwick.html.
McAll, R.K. (1981). *Healing the family tree*. London: Sheldon Press.
McGrath, A. (2002). *The reenchantment of nature: The denial of religion and the crises of ecology*. New York: Galilee.
McGuire, M.B. (1982). *Pentecostal Catholics*. Philadelphia: Temple University.
McGuire, M.B., & Kantor, D. (1998). *Ritual healing in suburban America*. New Brunswick, New Jersey: Rutgers
McHugh, P. R. (1993). "Multiple personality disorder." *Harvard Mental Health Letter*, *10*: 4-7.
McKanan, D. (2011). *Prophetic encounters: Religion and the American radical tradition*. Princeton: Beacon Press.
McNamara, D. (2015). "Chod." In *Spirit possession around the world: Possession, communion and demon expulsion across cultures*. Ed. J.P. Laycock. Pp. 83-85. Santa Barbara: ABC-CLIO.
MacNutt, F. (2009). *Deliverance from evil spirits: A practical guide*. Grand Rapids, MI: Chosen Books.
Manchester, W. (1993). *A world lit only by fire: The medieval mind and the Renaissance: A portrait of an age*. New York: Little, Brown and Company.

Martin, M. (1976). *Hostage to the devil: The possession and exorcism of five contemporary Americans*. New York: Reader's Digest: Thomas Y. Crowell Company.

—. (1987). *The Jesuits: The society of Jesus and the betrayal of the Roman Catholic Church*. New York: Simon and Schuster.

Marino, G.D. (2001). *Kierkegaard in the modern age*. Milwaukee: Marquette University Press.

Marlowe, C. (1604, 1994). *The tragical history of Doctor Faustus*. New York: Dover.

Marty, M.E. (2000). "Fundamentalism." In *Contemporary American religion*. Ed. W.C. Roof. Pp. 271-273. New York: MacMillan.

Matthews, W. (1995). *World religions, 2nd* ed. Minneapolis/St. Paul: West Publishing.

May, R. (1970). "Psychotherapy and the daimonic." In *Myths, dreams and religion*. Ed. J. Campbell. Pp. 196-211. Dallas, TX: Spring Books.

Mays, D. (2008). *The personality disorders*. Madison, WI: Clinicians Update.

McLaine, S. (1985). *Dancing in the light*. New York: Bantam.

Mehl-Madrona, L. *(2003). Coyote Healing: Miracles in native healing*. Rochester, VT: Bear & Co.

—. *(2008). Coyote wisdom: The power of story in healing*. Rochester, VT: Bear & Co.

Menghi, G., & Paxia, G. (2002). *The Devil's Scourge: Exorcism during Renaissance Italy*. Boston: Weiser.

Meigs, J.T. (1977). "Pastoral care methods and demonology in selected writings." *Journal of Psychology and Theology, 5*, 234-246.

Meggitt, J. (2015). "Antiquity." In *Spirit possession around the world: Possession, communion and demon expulsion across cultures*. Ed. J.P. Laycock. Pp. 17-19. Santa Barbara: ABC-CLIO.

Mercer, S. (Producer) & Shyamalan, M.N (Director). (2004). *The village* [Motion Picture]. USA: Touchstone.

Messing, S.D. (1967). "Group therapy and social status in the Zar cult of Ethiopia." In *Magic, witchcraft & curing*. Ed. J. Middleton. Pp. 285-293. Austin: University of Texas.

Middleton, J. (1967). "The concept of 'bewitching' in Lugbara." In *Magic, witchcraft & curing*. Ed. J. Middleton. Pp. 55-68. Austin: University of Texas.

Midelfort, H.C.E. (2005). *Exorcism and enlightenment: Johann Joseph Gassner and the demons of eighteenth-century Germany*. New Haven: Yale University Press.

Mikles, N.L. (2015a). “Kagura.” In *Spirit possession around the world: Possession, communion and demon expulsion across cultures*. Ed. J.P. Laycock. Pp. 197. Santa Barbara: ABC-CLIO.

—. (2015b). “Miko.” In *Spirit possession around the world: Possession, communion and demon expulsion across cultures*. Ed. J.P. Laycock. Pp. 236. Santa Barbara: ABC-CLIO.

—. (2015c). “Storytelling and spirit possession. In *Spirit possession around the world: Possession, communion and demon expulsion across cultures*. Ed. J.P. Laycock. Pp. 328-329. Santa Barbara: ABC-CLIO.

Miles, M. (2005). “Martin Luther and childhood disability in 16th century Germany: What did he write? What did he say? *Journal of Religion, Disability and Health*, 5 *(4)*: 5-36.

Miller, D. (1995). *Women hurt themselves: A book of hope and understanding*. New York: Basic Books.

Mischel, W., & Mischel, F. (1958). “Psychological aspects of spirit possession.” *American Anthropologist*, *60*, 249-260.

Modestino, E.J., & Halloran, C.S. (2015). “Michel, Anneliese.” In *Spirit possession around the world: Possession, communion and demon expulsion across cultures*. Ed. J.P. Laycock. Pp. 233-235. Santa Barbara: ABC-CLIO.

Monk, G., Winslade, J., Crocket, K., & Epston, D. (1997). *Narrative therapy in practice: The archaeology of hope*. San Francisco: John Wiley & Sons.

Monter, W. (2015). “Gordet, Dominic.” In *Spirit possession around the world: Possession, communion and demon expulsion across cultures*. Ed. J.P. Laycock. Pp. 63-67. Santa Barbara: ABC-CLIO.

Morehead, J.W. (2015a). “Johnson, Arne Cheyenne.” In *Spirit possession around the world: Possession, communion and demon expulsion across cultures*. Ed. J.P. Laycock. Pp. 189-190. Santa Barbara: ABC-CLIO.

—. (2015b). “Warren, Ed and Lorraine.” In *Spirit possession around the world: Possession, communion and demon expulsion across cultures*. Ed. J.P. Laycock. Pp. 366-369. Santa Barbara: ABC-CLIO.

—. (2015c). “Perron, Roger and Carolyn.” In *Spirit possession around the world: Possession, communion and demon expulsion across cultures*. Ed. J.P. Laycock. Pp. 284-285. Santa Barbara: ABC-CLIO.

—. (2015d). “Ramsey, Bill.” In *Spirit possession around the world: Possession, communion and demon expulsion across cultures*. Ed. J.P. Laycock. Pp. 299. Santa Barbara: ABC-CLIO.

Morris, I. (2011). *Why the west rules–for now: The patterns of history and what they reveal about the future.* New York: Picador.

Morrison, T. (1987). *Beloved*. New York: Vintage.

Moses, P. (2009). *The saint and the sultan: The crusades, Islam, and Francis of Assisi's mission of peace*. New York: Doubleday.

Moss, C. (2013). *The myth of persecution: How early Christians invented a story of martyrdom*. New York: HarperCollins.

Mott, M. (1993). *The seven mountains of Thoman Merton*. San Diego: Harvest.

Moyano, O., Claudon, P., Colin, V., Syatos, J., & Thiébaut, E. (2001). "Study of dissociative disorders and depersonalization in a sample of young adult French population," (article in French). *Encephale, 27 (6)*: 559-569.

Murakami, H. (1995). *The wind-up bird chronicles*. New York: Vintage.

Murguia, S.J. (2015). "Japanese new religious movements." In *Spirit possession around the world: Possession, communion and demon expulsion across cultures*. Ed. J.P. Laycock. Pp. 185-187. Santa Barbara: ABC-CLIO

Murphy, K.J. (2015a). "Abimelch." In *Spirit possession around the world: Possession, communion and demon expulsion across cultures*. Ed. J.P. Laycock. Pp. 1-2. Santa Barbara: ABC-Clio.

—. (2015b). "Azazel." In *Spirit possession around the world: Possession, communion and demon expulsion across cultures*. Ed. J.P. Laycock. Pp. 24-26. Santa Barbara: ABC-Clio.

Murray, D. (2015). *Personal communication*. June 26, 2015.

Muske-Dukes, C. (2008). *Channeling Mark Twain*. New York: Random House.

Nabokov, V. (2003). "An introductory essay." In *The strange case of Dr. Jekyll and Mr. Hyde*. New York: Signet Classics.

Nakatani, Y. (2000). "Dissociative disorders: From Janett to DSM-IV" [article in Japanese]. *Seishin Shinkeigaku Zasshi, 102 (1)*: 1-12.

Nakken, K.O., & Brodtkorb, E. (2011). "Epilepsy and religion" [article in Norwegian]. *Tidsskrift for den Norske laegeforen: tidsskrift for praktisk medicin, ny raekke, 131 (13-14)*: 1294-1297.

Nash, M. (1967). "Witchcraft as social process in Tzeltal community." In *Magic, witchcraft & curing*. Ed. J. Middleton. Austin: Texas University Press.

National Institute on Drug Abuse. (2014). "Treatment and recovery." Retrieved on October 26, 2016 from: https://www.drugabuse.gov/publications/drugs-brains-behavior-science-addiction/treatment-recovery.

Natoli, J. (1994). *Hauntings: Popular films and American culture: 1990-1992*. Albany, NY: State University of New York Press.

Neitz, M.J. (1987). *Charisma and Community*. New Brunswick, N.J.: Transaction.

Neki, J.S., Joinet, B., Ndosi, N., Kilonzo, G., Hauli, J.G., & Duvinage, G. (1986). "Witchcraft and psychotherapy." *British Journal of Psychiatry*, *149*: 145-155.

Nelson, V. (2012). *Gothicka*: *Vampire heroes, human gods and the new supernatural*. Cambridge, NJ: Harvard University Press.

Neuner, F., Pfeiffer, A., Schauer-Kaiser, E., Odenwald, M., Elbert, T., & Ertl, V. (2012). "Haunted by ghosts: prevalence, predictors and outcomes of spirit possession experiences among former child soldiers and war-affected civilians in Northern Uganda." *Social Science & Medicine*, *75 (3)*: 548-554.

Nevius, J.L. (1894*). Demon possession and allied themes*: *Being an inductive study of phenomena of our own times*. New York: Revel. Retrieved on February 16, 2016 from: https://archive.org/details/demonpossessiona00nevi.

Newell, L.F. (2015). "Trepanation." In *Spirit possession around the world*: *Possession, communion and demon expulsion across cultures*. Ed. J.P. Laycock. Pp. 352-353. Santa Barbara: ABC-CLIO.

News.Adventist. (undated). "Adventists not involved in reported exorcism in France." Retrieved on May 27, 2015 from: http://news.adventist.org/all-news/news/go/2013-10 10/adventists-not-involved-in-reported-exorcism-incident-in-france/.

Newberg, A. (2012). *The spiritual brain*: *Science and religious experience*. Chantilly, VA: The Teaching Company.

Nicole, D.F., & Manolache, C.M. (2015). "Tanacu exorcism." In *Spirit possession around the world*: *Possession, communion and demon expulsion across cultures*. Ed. J.P. Laycock. Pp. 332-334. Santa Barbara: ABC-CLIO.

Niebuhr, H.R. (1962, 1999). *The responsible self*. Westminster: John Knox Press.

Nolan, A. (1989). *Jesus before Christianity*. Maryknoll, NY: Orbis.

Noll, M.A. (2000). "Evangelical Christianity." In *Contemporary American religion*. Ed. W.C. Roof. Pp. 236-240. New York: MacMillan.

Norris, K. (1997). *The cloister walk*. New York: Riverhead.

—. (2001). *Dakota*: *A spiritual geography*. New York: Mariner.

—. (2008). *Acedia & me*: *A marriage, monks, and a writer's life*. New York: Riverhead Books.

Obeid, T., Abulaban, A., Al-Ghatani, F., Al-Malki, A.R., & Al-Ghamdi, A. (2012). "Possession by 'Jinn' as a cause of epilepsy (Saraa): A study from Saudi Arabia." *Seizure*, *21 (4)*: 245-249.

Oesterreich, T. (1930). *Possession: Demonical and other*. London: Kegan Paul.

Ofshe, R., & Watters, E. (1994). *Making monsters: False memories, psychotherapy and sexual hysteria*. Berkeley, CA: University of California Press.

Ogden, D. (2002). *Magic, witchcraft and ghosts in the Greek and Roman worlds: A sourcebook*. Oxford: Oxford University Press.

Ong, A. (1987). *Spirits of resistance and capitalist discipline: Factory women in Malaysia*. Albany: State University of New York Press.

Padoan, T. (2015). "Buddhism." In *Spirit possession around the world: Possession, communion and demon expulsion across cultures*. Ed. J.P. Laycock. Pp. 54-59. Santa Barbara: ABC-Clio.

Page, S.H.T. (1989). "The role of exorcism in clinical practice and pastoral care". *Journal of Psychology and Theology*, *17*, 121-131.

Pagels, E. (1996). *The origin of Satan: How Christianity demonized the Jews, pagans and heretics*. New York: Vintage.

Pardun, C.J. (1995). "Strange bedfellows: Symbols of religion and sexuality on MTV." *Youth Society*, *26 4*: 438-449.

Parry, A., & Doan, R.E. (1994). *Story re-vision: Narrative therapy in the postmodern world*. New York: Guilford.

Pasternak, J. (1988). "Obituaries: Father Karl Patzelt, 71, performed exorcisms." *Los Angeles Times*, May 23, 1988. Retrieved on March 11, 2016 from:
http://articles.latimes.com/1988-05-23/news/mn-2015_1_exorcisms.

Patterson, S. J. (2014). *The lost way: How two forgotten Gospels are rewriting the story of Christian origins*. New York: HarperOne.

Pattison, E.M., & Casey, R.L. (1969). "Glossolalia: A contemporary mystical experience." In *Clinical psychiatry and religion*. Pp. 133-148. New York: Little, Brown.

Pattison, E.M. (1973). "Exorcism and psychotherapy: A case of collaboration." In *Religious systems and psychotherapy*. Springfield, IL: Charles C. Thomas.

Peck, M.S. (1998). *People of the lie: The hope for healing human evil*. New York: Touchstone.

—. (2005). *Glimpses of the devil: A psychiatrist's personal accounts of possession, exorcism and redemption*. New York: Free Press.

Pendergrast, M. (2010). "Mark Pendergrast wraps up the *Inside the Outbreaks* book club." *The Science Blogs Book Club*. Retrieved on March 3, 2016 from:
http://scienceblogs.com/bookclub/2010/07/21/mark-pendergrast-wraps-up-the-1/.

Peretti, F.E. (2003). *Paretti Three Pack: This present darkness; Piercing the darkness, The prophet*. New York: Living Books.

Perriere, B.B., & Rozenberg, R. (2015). "Burma." In *Spirit possession around the world: Possession, communion and demon expulsion across cultures*. Ed. J.P. Laycock. Pp. 59-61. Santa Barbara: ABC-Clio.

Peterson, J.H. (1997). *The testament of Solomon*. Trans. F.C. Conybeare. Retrieved from http://www.esotericarchives.com/solomon/testamen.htm on January 27, 2016.

Peters, E. (2004). *Europe and the middle ages*. 4th ed. Upper Saddle River, NJ: Pearson.

Phillips, S.E. (2015a). "Baptism." In *Spirit possession around the world: Possession, communion and demon expulsion across cultures*. Ed. J.P. Laycock. Pp. 33-35. Santa Barbara: ABC-CLIO.

—. (2015b). "Catholicism." In *Spirit possession around the world: Possession, communion and demon expulsion across cultures*. Ed. J.P. Laycock. Pp. 63-67. Santa Barbara: ABC-CLIO.

—. (2015c.) "Gay, Antoine." In *Spirit possession around the world: Possession, communion and demon expulsion across cultures*. Ed. J.P. Laycock. Pp. 129-131. Santa Barbara: ABC-CLIO.

—. (2015d). "Martin, Malachi." In *Spirit possession around the world: Possession, communion and demon expulsion across cultures*. Ed. J.P. Laycock. Pp. 227-229. Santa Barbara: ABC-CLIO.

Piedmont, R.L., Village, A., & Dein, S. (1987). "Magic and jinn among Bangladeshis in the United Kingdom suffering from physical and mental health problems: controlling the uncontrollable." In *Research in the Social Scientific Study of Religion (Volume 24)*. Eds. R.L. Piedmont & A. Village. Pp. 193-220. Leiden, Netherlands: Brill.

Pipher, M. (2003). *Letters to a young therapist*. New York: Basic Books.

Plato. (1997). *Plato: The complete works*. New York: Hackett Publishing.

Pollen, J.H. (1912). "William Weston." *The Catholic Encyclopedia*. Retrieved on February 5, 2016 from: https://en.wikisource.org/wiki/Catholic_Encyclopedia_(1913)/William_Weston.

Poole, W.S. (2015). "Highgate cemetery." In *Spirit possession around the world: Possession, communion and demon expulsion across cultures.* Ed. J.P. Laycock. Pp. 141-143. Santa Barbara: ABC-CLIO.

Porter, R. (2002). *Madness: A brief history*. Oxford, UK: Oxford University Press.

Possamai, A. (2015). "Sociological interpretations." In *Spirit possession around the world: Possession, communion and demon expulsion across cultures.* Ed. J.P. Laycock. Pp. 317-320. Santa Barbara: ABC-CLIO.

Potok, C. *Wanderings: Chaim Potok's history of the Jews*. New York: Knopf.

Prest, J.G. (2011). *Anneliese: The exorcist tapes* [Motion Picture]. USA: Asylum.

Prince, R. (1966). *Trance and possession states*. Montreal: R.M. Bucke Memorial Society.

Prothero, S. (2010). *God is not one: The eight rival religions that run the world–and why their differences matter*. New York: HarperCollins.

Pullman, P. (1995). *The golden compass*. New York: Scholastic.

—. (1997). *The subtle knife*. New York: Scholastic.

—. (2000). *The amber spyglass*. New York: Scholastic.

Putman, F.W. (1985). "Dissociation as a response to extreme trauma." In *Childhood antecedents to multiple personality*. Ed. R.P. Klupf. Pp. 66-97. Washington, DC: APA Press.

Putz, U. (Producer) & Schmid, H.C. (2006). *Requiem* [Motion Picture]. Germany: 23/5 Filmproduktion GmbH Arte.

Pye, M. (2014). *The edge of the world: A cultural history of the North Sea and the transformation of Europe*. New York: Pegasus.

Quebedeaux, R. (1983). *The new charismatics II*. New York: Harper & Row.

RadioLab. (2007). "Crossroads", Retrieved on November 6, 2014 from: http://www.radiolab.org/story/199705-crossroads/.

Radl, K. (2012). "Jews, witches and Montague Summers." *Semite Controversies*. Retrieved on February 18, 2016 from: http://semiticcontroversies.blogspot.com/2012/08/jews-witches-and-montague-summers.html.

Rankine, C. (2015). "The New Review Q and A". *The Guardian*: 12/28/15.

Reece, E. (2016). *Utopia drive: A road trip through America's most radical idea*. New York: Farrar, Strauss & Giroux.

Reid, M. (2012). "Grandmother's footsteps: With no sign of a Cuban spring, change will have to come from within the party." *The Economist. Revolution in retreat, 8777*, 9-10.

Reis, R. (2013). "Children enacting idioms of witchcraft and spirit possession as a response to trauma: Therapeutically beneficial, and for whom?" *Transcultural Psychiatry*, *50 (5)*: 622-643.

Richardson, B.G., & Surmitis, K.A. (2014). "Responding to the rise in self-injury among youth." *Counseling Today*, *57 5*: 40-45.

Richardson, J.T., Best, J., & Bromley, D.G. (1991). *The Satanism scare*. New York: Aldine.
Rieber, R (1998). "Hypnosis, false memory and multiple personality: a trinity of affinity". *History of Psychiatry 10*, *37*: 3-11.
Robertson, P. (2003). *Bring it on*. Nashville, TN: W Publishing Group.
Rohr, R. (2007). *The little way*: *A spirituality of imperfection*. Albuquerque, NM: Center for Contemplation and Action.
Rokeach, M. (1960). *The open and closed mind*. New York: Basic Books.
Rosado, R.Q. (2010). *Consciousness-in-action*: *Toward an integral psychology of liberation and transformation*. Cagues, Puerto Rico: Ile.
Rosik, C.H. (1997). "When discernment fails: The case for outcome studies on exorcism." *Journal of Psychology and Theology*, *25*, 354-363.
—. (2003). "Critical issues in the dissociative disorders field: Six perspectives from religious sensitive practitioners." *Journal of Psychology and Theology*, *31*, 113-128.
Ross, C.A. (2011). "Possession experiences in dissociative identity disorder: A preliminary study." *Journal of Trauma and Dissociation*, *12 (4)*: 393-400.
Ross, C.A., Schroeder, E., & Ness, L. (2013). "Dissociation and symptoms of culture-bound syndromes in North America: A preliminary study." *Journal of Trauma and Dissociation*, *14 (2)*: 224-235.
Rothman, S. (1996). "Is God really dead in Beverly Hills?" *American Scholar*, *Spring*, 272-278.
Rubenstein, R.E. (2003). *Aristotle's children*: *How Christians, Muslims, and Jews rediscovered ancient wisdom and illuminated the Middle Ages*. Orlando, CA: Harvest.
Ruickbie, L. (2012). "'Child witches', from imaginary cannibalism to ritual abuse in London. *Paraanthropology*, *3 (3)*: 13-21.
—. (2015a). "The bell witch." In *Spirit possession around the world*: *Possession, communion and demon expulsion across cultures*. Ed. J.P. Laycock. Pp. 35-37. Santa Barbara: ABC-CLIO.
—. (2015b). "Hunkler, Ronald E." In *Spirit possession around the world*: *Possession, communion and demon expulsion across cultures*. Ed. J.P. Laycock. Pp. 156-158. Santa Barbara: ABC-CLIO.
—. (2015c). "Taylor, Michael." In *Spirit possession around the world*: *Possession, communion and demon expulsion across cultures*. Ed. J.P. Laycock. Pp. 337-339. Santa Barbara: ABC-CLIO.
Russell, G. (2014). *Heirs to Forgotten Kingdoms*: *Journey into disappearing religions of the Middle East*. New York: Basic.
Russell, J.B. (1972). *Witchcraft in the middle ages*. Ithaca, NY: Cornell University Press.

—. (1977). *The devil: Perceptions of evil of antiquity to primitive Christianity*. Ithaca, NY: Cornell University Press.

Ryan, B. (2017). "Christianity and mental health: Theology, activities, potential". Retrieved on 7/5/17 from: http://www.theosthinktank.co.uk/files/files/Christianity%20and%20Mental%20health%20WEB%20VERSION(1).pdf.

Sachs, O. (1999). *Migraines: The evolution of a common disorder*. New York: Vintage.

Sagert, K.B. (2015a). "Auma, Alice." In *Spirit possession around the world: Possession, communion and demon expulsion across cultures*. Ed. J.P. Laycock. Pp. 21-22. Santa Barbara: ABC-CLIO.

—. (2015b). "Talby, Dorothy." In *Spirit possession around the world: Possession, communion and demon expulsion across cultures*. Ed. J.P. Laycock. Pp. 331-332. Santa Barbara: ABC-CLIO.

Saler, B. (1967). "Nagual, witch, and sorcerer in a Quiché village." In *Magic, witchcraft, & curing*. Ed. J. Middleton. Pp. 69-99. Austin: University of Texas Press.

Salie, F. (2016). *Approval junkie: Adventures in caring too much*. Crown Archetype: New York.

Salzman, M. (2001). *Lying awake*. New York: Vintage.

Salzmann, A.B. (2015). "Rituale romanum." In *Spirit possession around the world: Possession, communion and demon expulsion across cultures*. Ed. J.P. Laycock. Pp. 300-303. Santa Barbara: ABC-CLIO.

Sapkota, R.P., Gurung, D., Neupane, D., Shah, S.K., Kienzler, H., & Kirmayer, L.J. (2014). "A village possessed by 'witches': a mixed-methods case-control study of possession and common mental disorders in rural Nepal." *Culture, Medicine & Psychiatry, 38 (4)*: 642-668.

Sar, V., Alioğlu, F., Akyüz, G. (2014). "Experiences of possession and paranormal phenomena among women in the general population: Are they related to traumatic stress and dissociation?" *Journal of Trauma Dissociation, 15 (3)*; 303-18.

Sar, V., Yargic, L.I., & Tutkun, H. (1996). "Structured interview data on 35 cases of dissociative identity disorder in Turkey." *American Journal of Psychiatry, 153 (10)*: 1329-1333.

Sar, U., Unal, S.N., Kizilton, E. (2001). "HMPAO Spect study of cerebral perfusion in dissociative identity disorder." *Journal of Trauma Dissociation, 5*, 5-25.

Satir, V. (1964). *Conjoint family therapy*. Palo Alto, CA: Science and Behavior Books.

Satoh, S., Obata, S., Seno, E., Okada, T., Morita, N., Saito, T., Yoshikawa, M., Yamagami, A. (1996). "A case of possessive state with onset influenced by 'door-to-door' sales." *Psychiatry and Clinical Neurosciences, 50 (6)*: 313-316.

Saunders, W. P. (2003). "St. Michael the Archangel." *Arlington Catholic Herald*. Retrieved on October 31, 2014 from: http://www.catholicherald.com/stories/St-Michael-the-Archangel,3401?content_source=&category_id=&search_filter=Saunders+2003&event_mode=&event_ts_from=&list_type=&order_by=&order_sort=&content_class=&sub_type=stories,blogs&town_id=.

Sawgi, M. (2015). "Sudan's great depression: Mental illness dangerously ignored by country's health services." Retrieved on October 26, 2016 from: http://africanarguments.org/2015/04/08/sudans-great-depression-mental-illness-dangerously-ignored-by-countrys-health-services-by-dr-mohamed-shawgi/.

Schenk, R. (2001). *The sunken quest, the wasted fisher, the pregnant fish: Postmodern reflections on modern depth psychology*. Wilmette, IL: Chiron.

Schmidt, B.E. (2015a). "Afro-Atlantic religions." In *Spirit possession around the world: Possession, communion and demon expulsion across cultures*. Ed. J.P. Laycock. Pp. 2-6. Santa Barbara: ABC-CLIO.

—. (2015b). "Gender." In *Spirit possession around the world: Possession, communion and demon expulsion across cultures*. Ed. J.P. Laycock. Pp. 133-135. Santa Barbara: ABC-CLIO.

Scull, A. (2015). *Madness in civilization: A cultural history of insanity from the Bible to Freud, from the madhouse to modern medicine*. Princeton: Princeton University Press.

Scull, D. (2012). *Hysteria: The disturbing history*. Oxford: Oxford University Press.

Sersch, M. (2013). "Demons on the couch: Spirit possession, exorcism and dissociative trance disorder." *Journal of Exceptional Experiences in Psychology, 1*: 11-17.

Shakespeare, W. (2005). *The Oxford Shakespeare*. Oxford: Oxford University Press.

Shapiro, L. (2016). "Miracles–or not?" *Wisconsin Public Radio University of the Air*. Retrieved on August 1, 2016 from: http://www.wpr.org/shows/miracles-%E2%80%94-or-not.

Shekar, C.R.C. (1989). "Possession syndrome in India." In *Altered states of consciousness and mental health: A cross-cultural perspective*. Ed. C. Ward. Newbury Park: Sage Publications.

Shermer, M. (2003). "Demon-haunted brain: If the brain mediates all experiences, then paranormal phenomena are nothing more than neuronal events." *Scientific American, 28 (3)*: 25.

Sherwood, H. (2017). "'Spiritual abuse': Christian thinktank warns of sharp rise in UK exorcisms." Retrieved on 7/5/17 from: https://www.theguardian.com/world/2017/jul/05/christian-thinktank-warns-of-rise-in-exorcisms-mental-health.

Showalter, E. (1997). *Hystories: Hysterical epidemics and modern culture*. London: Doubleday.

Siezmore, C., & Pittillo, E. (1977). *I'm Eve*. Garden City, NY: Doubleday.

Sigelman, C.K., & Rider, E.A. (2007). *Life-span human development*. 6th edition. Belmont, CA: Wadsworth Cengage.

Smith, D. (1982). "The metaphor of race in American literature." *Berkshire Review*, 62-64.

Snopes. (2011). "KISS: Does it stand for Knights in satanic service?" Retrieved on September 27, 2016 from: http://www.snopes.com/music/hidden/kiss.asp.

Soloman, A. (2002). *The noonday demon: An atlas of depression*. New York: Scribner.

Somasundaram, D., Thivakaran, T., & Bhugra, D. (2008). "Possession states in Northern Sri Lanka." *Psychopathology*, *41 (4)*: 245-253.

Spanos, N.E., Menary, E., Gaboram N., DuBreuil, S., & Dewhirst, B. (1991). "Secondary identity enactments during hypnotic past-life regression: A socio-cognitive perspective." *Journal of Personality and Social Psychology*, *61*, 308-320.

Spiegel, D., Lewis-Fernández, R., Lanuis, R., Vermetten, E., Simeon, D., & Friedman, M. (2013). "Dissociative disorders in DSM-5." *Annual Review of Clinical Psychology*, *9*: 299-326.

Spiegel, D., Loewenstein, R.L., Lewis- Fernández, R., Sar, V., Simeon, D., Vermetten, E., Cardeña, E., Dell, P.F. (2011). "Dissociative disorders in the DSM-5." *Depression and Anxiety*, *28 9*: 824-852.

Spiro, H. (1998). *The power of hope: A doctor's perspective*. New Haven: Yale University Press.

Spiro, N. (1967). *Burmese supernaturalism: A study into the explanation and reduction of suffering*. Englewood Cliffs, NJ: Prentice-Hall.

Spong, J.S. (1994). *Resurrection: Myth or reality: A Bishop's search for the origins of Christianity*. San Francisco: Harper.

Stalker, M. (Director) & Marro, R. (Producer). (2016). *Hostage to the devil* [Motion picture]. Ireland: Causeway Pictures.

Starr, P. (1984). *The social transformation of American medicine: The rise of a sovereign profession and the making of a vast industry*. New York: Basic.

Stein, D.J., Koenen, K.C., Friedman, M.J., Hill, E., McLaughlin, K.A., Petukhova, M., Shahly, V., Spiegel, D., Borges, G., Bunting, B., Caldasde-Almeida, J.M., de Girolman, G., Demyttenaere, K., Florescu, S., Haro, J.M., Karam, E.G., Kovess-Masfety, V., Lee, S., Matchinger, H., Mladenova, M., Posada-Villa, J., Tachimori, H., Viana, M.C., & Kessler, R.C. (2013). "Dissociation in posttraumatic stress disorder: Evidence from the world mental health surveys." *Biological Psychiatry, 73 (4)*: 302-312.

Stephens, W. (2002). *Demon lovers: Witchcraft, sex, and the crisis of belief.* Chicago: University of Chicago Press.

Stevens, P., & Smith, R.L. (2009). *Substance abuse counseling: Theory and practice*. 4th ed. Upper Saddle River, New Jersey: Pearson.

Stevenson, K. (2007*). Rooted in detachment: Living the transfiguration.* Collegeville, MN: Cistercian Studies.

Stevenson, R.L. (1886/2003). *The strange case of Dr. Jekyll and Mr. Hyde.* New York: Signet Classics.

Stoller, P., & Olkes, C. (1987). *In sorcery's shadow: A memoir of apprenticeship among the Songay of Niger*. Chicago: University of Chicago Press.

Stoller, P. (1989). *Fusion of worlds: An ethnography of possession among the Songay of Niger*. Chicago: University of Chicago Press.

Straussner, S.L.A. (2001). *Ethnocultural factors in substance abuse treatment*. New York: Guilford.

Substance Abuse and Mental Health Services Administration. (2007). *Substance abuse treatment for persons with co-occurring disorders in-service training: Based upon a treatment improvement protocol TIP 42*. Rockville, MD: U.S. Department of Health and Human Services.

—. (2014). *Improving cultural competence, TIP 59*. Rockville, MD: U.S. Department of Health and Human Services.

—. (2015). *Core competencies for peer workers in behavioral health services*. Rockville, MD: U.S. Department of Health and Human Services.

Summers, M. (1926). *History of witchcraft and demonology*. London: Routledge.

—. (1958). *Geography of witchcraft*. New York: Sheed and Ward.

Tahir, T. (2005). "'My exorcisms get results' says voodoo priest of North London." *Telegraph*. 19 June 2005. Retrieved on November 1, 2016 from: http://www.telegraph.co.uk/news/uknews/1492346/My-exorcisms-get-results-says-voodoo-priest-of-north-London.html.

Tajima-Pozo, K., Zambrano-Enriques, D., de Anta, L., Moron, M.D., Carrasco, J.L., Lopez-Ibor, J.J., & Diaz-Marasa, M. (2005). "Practicing exorcism in schizophrenia." *Medical Anthropology (24), 2*: 111-144.

Tallis, R. (2011). *Aping mankind: Neuromania, darwinitis, and the misrepresentation of humanity*. New York: Acumen Press.

Taylor, C. (2007). *A secular age*. Cambridge, MA: Belknap.

Teague, M. (2016). "Clown sightings: The day it all began." *The Guardian*. Retrieved on October 6, 2016 from: https://www.theguardian.com/culture/2016/oct/05/clown-sightings-south-carolina-alabama?utm_source=esp&utm_medium=Email&utm_campaign=GU+Today+USA+-+morning+briefing+2016&utm_term=193667&subid=14329163&CMP=ema_a-morning-briefing_b-morning-briefing_c-US_d-1.

Thigpen, C.H., & Cleckley, H.M. (1957). *The three faces of Eve*. New York: McGraw-Hill.

Thomas, K. (1971). *Religion and the Decline of Magic*. New York: Penguin.

Thomason, T.C. (2008). "Possession, exorcism and psychotherapy." Retrieved on March 6, 2017 from: http://www.shsu.edu/~piic/winter2008/Thomason.html.

Thompson, L.C. (2009). *William Scott Ament and the Boxer rebellion: Heroism, hubris and the ideal missionary*. Jefferson, NC: McFarland.

Tippet, K. (2012). *On being*. Retrieved on 8/6/12 from: http://www.onbeing.org/program/spiritual-boundariesmodern-turkey-fr-alberto ambrosio-and-metropolitan-elpidophoros.

Tippet, K. (2016). *On becoming wise: An inquiry into the mystery and art of living*. Audiobook. New York: Penguin Press.

Torrey, E.F. (1986). *Witchdoctors and psychiatrists: The common roots of psychiatry and its future*. New York: Perennial/Harper & Row.

Van der Kolk, B. (2014). *The body keeps the score: Brain, mind and body in the healing of trauma*. New York: Penguin.

Van Duijl, M., Cardeña, E., & de Jong, J. (2005). "The validity of DSM-IV dissociative disorders categories in south-west Uganda." *Transcultural Psychiatry*, *42 (2)*: 219-241.

Van Duijl, M., Kleijn, W., & de Jong, J. (2013). "Are symptoms of spirit possessed patients covered by the DSM-IV or DSM-5 criteria for possession trance disorder? A mixed method explorative study in Uganda." *Social Psychiatry and Psychiatric Epidemiology*, *48 (9)*: 1417-1730.

Van Duijl, M., Kleijn, W., & de Jong, J. (2014). "Unravelling the spirits' message: a study of help-seeking steps and explanatory models among patients suffering from spirit possession in Uganda." *International Journal of Mental Health Systems*, *8 (24)*. Retrieved on March 30, 2014 from: http://www.ncbi.nlm.nih.gov/pubmed/24940355.

van Duijl, M., Nijenhuis, E., Komroe, I.H., Gernaat, H.B., & de Jong, J. (2013). "Dissociative symptoms and reported trauma among patients with spirit possession and matched healthy controls in Uganda." *Journal of Trauma and Dissociation, 14 (2)*: 224-235.

Varlack, C.A. (2015). "Hurston, Zora Neale." In *Spirit possession around the world: Possession, communion and demon expulsion across cultures*. Ed. J.P. Laycock. Pp. 159-160. Santa Barbara: ABC-CLIO.

Vásquez, A.G. (2015). "Morocco." In *Spirit possession around the world: Possession, communion and demon expulsion across cultures*. Ed. J.P. Laycock. Pp. 243-244. Santa Barbara: ABC-CLIO.

Verter, B. (2000). "Devils, demons and spirits." In *Contemporary American religion*. Ed. W.C. Roof. Pp. 185-187. New York: MacMillan.

Vowell, S. (2009). *The wordy shipmates*. New York: Riverhead.

Wagner, C.P. (2011). *Spiritual warfare strategy: Confronting spiritual powers*. Shippensburg, PA: Destiny Image Books.

Wait, wait, don't tell me. (2014). Retrieved on 10/28, 2014 from: http://www.npr.org/programs/wait-wait-dont-tell-me/358567782/wait-wait-dont-tell-me-for-oct-25-2014.

Wald, E. (2004). *Escaping the delta: Robert Johnson and the invention of the blues*. New York: HarperCollins.

Wall, J.C. (1904). *Devils*. London: Methuen & Co.

Walsh, B.W. (2014). *Treating self-injury, 2nd ed*. New York: Guilford.

Walsh, B. W., & Rosen, P.M. (1988). *Self-mutilation: Theory, research and treatment*. New York: Guilford.

Ward, C. (1980). "Spirit possession and mental health: A psycho-anthropological perspective." *Human Relations, 33*: 149-163.

Ward, L. (1978). *God's man: A woodcut in novels*. New York: St. Martin's Press.

Watters, E. (2011). *Crazy like us: The globalization of the American psyche*. New York: Free Press.

Watson, C. (2015a). "Christine Watson on her novel 'Where women are kings'". *To the Best of Our Knowledge*, June 14, 2015. Retrieved on June 28, 2015 from: http://www.wnyc.org/story/christie-watson-on-her-novel-where-women-are-kings/.

—. (2015b). *Where women are kings*. New York: Other Press.

Waszynski, M. (Producer) & Mayflauer, Z. (Director). (1937). *The Dybbuk [Motion Picture]*. Poland: Warszawskie Biuro Kinematograficzbe Femiks.

Webb, J. (1976). *The occult establishment*. New York. Open Court Press.

Weeks, N.P. (1996). "Reconciling scientific and religious discourse about madness during the age of reason: Lessons for today?" *Journal of Psychiatric and Mental Health Nursing, 3 (2)*: 95-101.

Weiner, W. (2011). *Man seeks God: My flirtations with the Divine*. New York: 12 Books.

Weller, P.T. (1952). *The Roman ritual in Latin and English with rubrics and plainchant notation*. Volume 2. Milwaukee: Bruce Publishing.

Wellman, J. (2000). *Grassroots reform in the burned-over district of upstate New York: Religion, abolitionism and democracy*. London: Routledge.

Welwood, J. (2000). *Towards a psychology of awakening: Buddhism, psychotherapy and the path of personal and spiritual transformation*. Boston: Shambala.

Werse, N.R. (2015a). "Des Valles, Marie." In *Spirit possession around the world: Possession, communion and demon expulsion across cultures*. Ed. J.P. Laycock. Pp. 109-110. Santa Barbara: ABC-CLIO.

—. (2015b). "Glossolalia." In *Spirit possession around the world: Possession, communion and demon expulsion across cultures*. Ed. J.P. Laycock. Pp. 137-139. Santa Barbara: ABC-CLIO.

—. (2015c). "Loudan." In *Spirit possession around the world: Possession, communion and demon expulsion across cultures*. Ed. J.P. Laycock. Pp. 219-222. Santa Barbara: ABC-CLIO.

Westerbeck, C.L. (1974). "The banality of evil." *Commonweal*. March 1, 1974: 532-533.

Westerlink, H. (2014). "Demonic possession and the historical construct of hysteria and neurosis." *Historical Psychiatry, 25 (3)*: 335-49.

What's the harm website. (2015). Retrieved on March 12, 2015 from: http://whatstheharm.net/exorcisms.htm.

White, H. (2006). *Post-modernism 101: A first course for the curious Christian*. Grand River, MI: Brazos Press.

Wilkinson, K. (2015). "Anthony, St." In *Spirit possession around the world: Possession, communion and demon expulsion across cultures*. Ed. J.P. Laycock. Pp. 15-17. Santa Barbara: ABC-CLIO.

Wilkinson, T. (2007). *The Vatican's exorcists: Driving out the devil in the 21st century*. New York: Warner.

Williams, R.H. (2000). "Culture wars." In *Contemporary American religion*. Ed. W.C. Roof. Pp.165-166. New York: MacMillan.

Wilson-Hartgrove, J. (2008). *New monasticism: What it has to say to today's church*. Grand Rapids, MI: Brazos.

Winn, C.T.C. (2015a). "Blumhardt, Christoph Friedrich." In *Spirit possession around the world: Possession, communion and demons*. Ed. J.P. Laycock. Pp. 46-47. Santa Barbara: ABC CLIO.

—. (2015b). "Blumhardt, Johann Chritoph." In *Spirit possession around the world: Possession, communion and demons*. Ed. J.P. Laycock. Pp. 47-49. Santa Barbara: ABC CLIO.

Winzeler, R.L. (2012). *Anthropology and religion*. 2nd ed. Lanham, MD: AltaMira.

Wise, D. (2015). "Wagner, C. Peter." In *Spirit possession around the world: Possession, communion and demons*. Ed. J.P. Laycock. Pp. 365-366. Santa Barbara: ABC-CLIO.

Wiseman, T. (2016). "The truth about crystal meth, witchcraft and demons." Retrieved on February 8, 2016 from: http://hubpages.com/religion-philosophy/The-Truth-About-Meth--Witchcraft--And-Demons.

Wisse, F. (1988). "The apocryphon of John." In *The Nag Hammadi library: The definitive translation of the Gnostic scriptures complete in one volume*. Ed. J.M. Robinson. Pp.105-124. New York: HarperOne.

Wittgenstein, L. (1953). *Philosophic investigations*. New York: Blackwell.

Wolheim, P. (2014). "The case for animal-protective counseling practice." *Counseling Today 57, 5*: 47-50.

Wood, C. (2015a). "Korean shamanism." In *Spirit possession around the world*: *Possession, communion and demons*. Ed. J.P. Laycock. Pp. 207-210. Santa Barbara: ABC-CLIO.

—. (2015b). "Zar." In *Spirit possession around the world*: *Possession, communion and demons*. Ed. J.P. Laycock. Pp. 379-381. Santa Barbara: ABC-CLIO.

Woodward, K.L. (2016). *Getting religion*: *Faith, culture, and politics from the age of Eisenhower to the era of Obama*. New York: Convergent.

Woods, J. (2014). "Billy Milligan\1955-2014: Man with famous insanity plea dies." *The Columbus Dispatch*, December 17, 2014: retrieved on April 22, 2015 from: http://www.dispatch.com/content/stories/local/2014/12/16/1216-billy-milligan-dies.html.

Wuthnow, R. (1988). *The restructuring of American religion*: *Society and faith since World War II*. Princeton, NJ: Princeton University Press.

Yalom, I. (1989). *Love's executioner and other tales of psychotherapy*. New York: Basic.

Yonchak, M. (2015). "Music, popular." In *Spirit possession around the world*: *Possession, communion and demons*. Ed. J.P. Laycock. Pp. 244-247. Santa Barbara: ABC-CLIO.

Young, S. (2018). *Women who fly*: *Goddesses, witches, mystics, and other airborn females*. Oxford: Oxford University Press.

Zitkala-Sa. (1921, 1985). *American Indian Stories*. Lincoln, NE: Bison Books.

Zoja, L. (1989). *Drugs, addiction and initiation*: *The modern search for ritual*. Trans. M.E. Romano & R. Mercurio. Boston: Sigo.

INDEX